NEW DEVELOPMENTS IN THE PATHOGENESIS OF RHEUMATOID ARTHRITIS

Edited by **Lazaros I. Sakkas**

New Developments in the Pathogenesis of Rheumatoid Arthritis
http://dx.doi.org/10.5772/63175
Edited by Lazaros I. Sakkas

Contributors

Reem Hamdy A Mohammed, Hesham Elmakhzangy, Victoria Sarafian, Maria Kazakova, Toshihiro Nakajima, Naoko Yagishita, Satoko Aratani, Hidetoshi Fujita, Yoshihisa Yamano, Kusuki Nishioka, Agnieszka Paradowska-Gorycka, Barbara Stypinska, Codrina Ancuta, Cristina Iordache, Eugen Ancuta, Mihailov Claudia, Selim Nalbant, Merih Birlik, Duygu Harmancı, Ayse Kocak, Daniela Opris, Cristina Pomirleanu

Published by InTech

Janeza Trdine 9, 51000 Rijeka, Croatia

Publishing Process Manager Iva Lipovic
Technical Editor SPi Global
Cover InTech Design team

First published February, 2017
Printed in Croatia
Legal deposit, Croatia: National and University Library in Zagreb

Additional hard copies can be obtained from orders@intechopen.com

New Developments in the Pathogenesis of Rheumatoid Arthritis, Edited by Lazaros I. Sakkas
p. cm.
Print ISBN 978-953-51-2969-1
Online ISBN 978-953-51-2970-7

For EU product safety concerns:
IN TECH d.o.o., Prolaz Marije Krucifikse Kozulić 3, 51000 Rijeka, Croatia,
info@intechopen.com or visit our website at intechopen.com.

Meet the editor

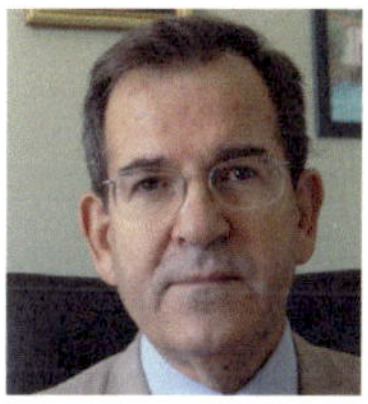

Lazaros I. Sakkas, MD, DM, PhD (UK), FRCP (UK), is a professor of internal medicine and rheumatology and chairman of the Department of Rheumatology and Clinical Immunology, Medical School, University of Thessaly. He is also an adjunct professor at the Old Dominion University, Norfolk, VA, USA. He did his PhD at Guy's Hospital, London, where he also trained in rheumatology, and then worked at the Ioannina Medical School, Ioannina, Greece, and at the Temple University Medical School, Philadelphia, PA, USA. His research focused on T cells, B cells, systemic sclerosis, osteoarthritis, and inflammatory arthritis. He has more than 105 publications and chapters in 8 books. He is the editor of Mediterranean Journal of Rheumatology and serves in editorial boards of some journals and as reviewer in many journals.

Contents

Preface

Rheumatoid arthritis (RA) is a systemic inflammatory disease characterized mainly by symmetrical polyarthritis. It affects more women than men, and early studies, based on the low concordance rate of RA in monozygotic twins but increased concordance rate relative to dizygotic twins, indicated a major role for environmental factors [1,2]. The etiopathogenesis of RA is not completely understood, but some pathogenetic aspects can be inferred from synovial histology, joint erosions, cytokines produced in the joints, and effects of targeted treatment. The synovial membrane in RA is characterized by heavy infiltration of T cells, B cells, and macrophages which frequently take the form of nodular, lymphoid-like ectopic structures, which are able to produce antibodies locally. In RA joints, there is production of pro-inflammatory cytokines, such as IL-12, TNF-α, IL-1b, IL-6, and IL-17. The clinical response to biological anticytokine agents, such as anti-TNF-α (adalimumab, etanercept, golimumab, remicade, and certolizumab pegol), anti–IL-6 (tocilizumab), and anti–IL-1 (anakinra), reinforces the pathogenic role of the respective cytokines in the pathogenesis of RA. The presence of autoantibodies, namely, rheumatoid factor and anticitrullinated peptide antibodies (ACPAs), classified RA as an autoimmune disease and implied a role for B cells in the pathogenesis of RA. Again, the effectiveness of anti–B-cell treatment with anti-CD20 monoclonal antibody (rituximab) reinforced the pathogenetic role of B cells in RA [3].

Among genetic factors, the HLA-DRB1 shared epitope (HLA-DRB1SE), a common amino acid sequence of the HLA-DR β chain of alleles positively associated with RA, such as HLA-DRB1*04:01, 04:04, 01:01, and 10:01, stands out as the most important genetic factor [4]. The detection of oligoclonal populations of T cells in RA joints suggested that T cells recognize antigens, and this finding fitted nicely with the HLA association of RA, since HLA molecules present antigenic peptides to T cells [5]. The effectiveness of CTLA-4-IgGFc treatment (abatacept) confirmed the pathogenetic role of T cells in RA. However, it was the discovery of ACPAs, which are present in around 70% of RA patients, that had a major impact on the elucidation of pathogenesis of RA. Citrullination is a posttranslational modification of proteins and is mediated by peptidylarginine deiminase (PAD), an enzyme that catalyzes the change of arginine residues into citrulline. Cigarette smoking, periodontitis, two environmental factors, and HLA-DRB1SE are major risk factors for RA, and this association is attributed to ACPA production [6]. In RA, HLA-DRB1SE preferentially binds to citrullinated peptides and presents these peptides to T cells [7,8], which in turn are activated and also provide help to B cells for differentiation and ACPA production. It appears that citrullination itself is key to T-cell recognition specificity, since crystal structure of HLADRB*04:01 complexed with α-enolase peptide or with its respective citrullinated peptide did not alter the conformation of the peptide [9]. Autophagy is involved in protein citrullination [10], and there is a significant association between levels of autophagy and ACPAs in early RA [11]. EBV infection through citrullination and molecular mimicry may also be involved. Epstein-Barr virus (EBV) antigens are recognized by T cells in RA joints [12,13], and antibodies to EBNA-derived citrullinated peptide are present in RA patients and cross-react with fibrin-derived citrullinated peptide [14], thus linking EBV infection with citrullination. Another source of citrullinated peptides is NETosis, the formation of neutrophil extracellular traps (NETs), which is a form of cell death to increase microbial killing. During NETosis, citrullination of core histones takes place. Furthermore, B cells from RA synovial membrane ectopic lymphoid structures target citrullinated histones from NETs [15].

Protein citrullination appears to cause arthritis in experimental arthritis models [6], and this has led to the introduction of immunotherapy with citrullinated peptide dendritic cells to RA patients carrying HLA-DRB1SE in a phase 1 study with encouraging results [16].

Epigenetics, which include DNA methylation, histone modification, and microRNAs, modify gene expression without changing gene DNA sequence and are involved in RA. DNA methylation aberrations are detected in RA [17,18], and DNA methylation at two particular sites was the stronger predictor of response to disease-modifying antirheumatic drugs in early RA [19].

Microbiota, a new area of research, revealed interesting influences on arthritis development. Altered microbiome composition has been documented in RA [20,21], and in mice, the gut microbiome has been found to influence susceptibility to collagen-induced arthritis [22]. Interestingly, HLA is associated with gut microbiome composition. The gut microbiome of transgenic mice carrying the RA-susceptible HLA-DRB1*04:01 was dominated by Clostridia-like species, whereas that of mice carrying the RA-resistant, HLA-DRB1*04:02 was dominated by bifidobacteria [23,24]. Furthermore, the presence of bifidobacteria was negatively correlated with Th17 cells in the gut [24].

In conclusion, it has become increasingly clear that citrullinated proteins are autoantigens in RA and that additional factors, such as epigenetic factors and gut microbiota, influence arthritis. In this book, various and novel pathogenetic aspects of RA are discussed in detail.

References

[1] Silman AJ, MacGregor AJ, Thomson W, Holligan S, Carthy D, Farhan A, Ollier WE. Twin concordance rates for rheumatoid arthritis: results from a nationwide study. Br J Rheumatol. 1993;32(10):903-7.

[2] Hensvold AH, Magnusson PK, Joshua V, Hansson M, Israelsson L, Ferreira R, Jakobsson PJ, Holmdahl R, Hammarström L, Malmström V, Askling J, Klareskog L, Catrina AI. Environmental and genetic factors in the development of anticitrullinated protein antibodies (ACPAs) and ACPA-positive rheumatoid arthritis: an epidemiological investigation in twins. Ann Rheum Dis. 2015;74:375-80

[3] Combe B, Landewe R, Daien CI, Hua C, Aletaha D, Álvaro-Gracia JM, Bakkers M, Brodin N, Burmester GR, Codreanu C, Conway R, Dougados M, Emery P, Ferraccioli G, Fonseca J, Raza K, Silva-Fernández L, Smolen JS, Skingle D, Szekanecz Z, Kvien TK, van der Helm-van Mil A, van Vollenhoven R. 2016 update of the EULAR recommendations for the management of early arthritis. Ann Rheum Dis. 2016, Dec 15. pii: annrheumdis-2016-210602. doi: 10.1136/annrheumdis-2016-210602. [Epub ahead of print]

[4] Wordsworth BP, Lanchbury JS, Sakkas LI, Welsh KI, Panayi GS, Bell JI. HLA-DR4 subtype frequencies in rheumatoid arthritis indicate that DRB1 is the major susceptibility locus within the HLA class II region. Proc Natl Acad Sci USA. 1989;86(24):10049-53.

[5] Sakkas LI, Chen PF, Platsoucas CD. T-cell antigen receptors in rheumatoid arthritis. Immunol Res. 1994;13(2-3):117-38.

[6] Sakkas LI, Bogdanos DP, Katsiari C, Platsoucas CD.Anti-citrullinated peptides as autoantigens in rheumatoid arthritis-relevance to treatment. Autoimmun Rev. 2014;13(11):1114-20.

[7] Hill JA, Southwood S, Sette A, Jevnikar AM, Bell DA, Cairns E. Cutting edge: the conversion of arginine to citrulline allows for a high-affinity peptide interaction with the rheumatoid arthritis-associated HLA-DRB1*0401 MHC class II molecule. J Immunol. 2003;171(2):538-41.

[8] Scally SW, Petersen J, Law SC, Dudek NL, Nel HJ, Loh KL, Wijeyewickrema LC, Eckle SB, van Heemst J, Pike RN, McCluskey J, Toes RE, La Gruta NL, Purcell AW, Reid HH, Thomas R, Rossjohn J. A molecular basis for the association of the HLA-DRB1 locus, citrullination, and rheumatoid arthritis. J Exp Med. 2013;210:2569-82.

[9] Gerstner C, Dubnovitsky A, Sandin C, Kozhukh G, Uchtenhagen H, James EA, Rönnelid J, Ytterberg AJ, Pieper J, Reed E, Tandre C, Rieck M, Zubarev RA, Rönnblom L, Sandalova T, Buckner JH, Achour A, Malmström V. Functional and Structural Characterization of a Novel HLA-DRB1*04:01-Restricted α-Enolase T Cell Epitope in Rheumatoid Arthritis. Front Immunol. 2016;7:494.

[10] Ireland JM, Unanue ER. Autophagy in antigen-presenting cells results in presentation of citrullinated peptides to CD4 T cells. J Exp Med. 2011;208(13):2625-32.

[11] Sorice M, Iannuccelli C, Manganelli V, Capozzi A, Alessandri C, Lococo E, Garofalo T, Di Franco M, Bombardieri M, Nerviani A, Misasi R, Valesini G. Autophagy generates citrullinated peptides in human synoviocytes: a possible trigger for anti-citrullinated peptide antibodies. Rheumatology (Oxford). 2016;55(8):1374-85.

[12] Tan LC, Mowat AG, Fazou C, Rostron T, Roskell H, Dunbar PR, Tournay C, Romagné F, Peyrat MA, Houssaint E, Bonneville M, Rickinson AB, McMichael AJ, Callan MF. Specificity of T cells in synovial fluid: high frequencies of CD8(+) T cells that are specific for certain viral epitopes. Arthritis Res. 2000;2(2):154-64.

[13] Croia C, Serafini B, Bombardieri M, Kelly S, Humby F, Severa M, Rizzo F, Coccia EM, Migliorini P, Aloisi F, Pitzalis C. Epstein-Barr virus persistence and infection of autoreactive plasma cells in synovial lymphoid structures in rheumatoid arthritis. Ann Rheum Dis. 2013 Sep 1;72(9):1559-68

[14] Toussirot E, Roudier J. Pathophysiological links between rheumatoid arthritis and the Epstein-Barr virus: an update. Joint Bone Spine. 2007;74(5):418-26.

[15] Corsiero E, Bombardieri M, Carlotti E1, Pratesi F, Robinson W, Migliorini P, Pitzalis C. Single cell cloning and recombinant monoclonal antibodies generation from RA synovial B cells reveal frequent targeting of citrullinated histones of NETs. Ann Rheum Dis. 2016;75(10):1866-75.

[16] Benham H, Nel HJ, Law SC, Mehdi AM, Street S, Ramnoruth N, Pahau H, Lee BT, Ng J, Brunck ME, Hyde C, Trouw LA, Dudek NL, Purcell AW, O'Sullivan BJ, Connolly JE, Paul SK, Lê Cao KA, Thomas R. Citrullinated peptide dendritic cell immunotherapy in HLA risk genotype-positive rheumatoid arthritis patients. Sci Transl Med. 2015;7(290):290ra87.

[17] Glossop JR, Emes RD, Nixon NB, Packham JC, Fryer AA, Mattey DL, Farrell WE. Genome-wide profiling in treatment-naive early rheumatoid arthritis reveals DNA methylome changes in T and B lymphocytes. Epigenomics. 2016;8(2):209-24.
[18] Gomez-Cabrero D, Almgren M, Sjöholm LK, Hensvold AH, Ringh MV, Tryggvadottir R, Kere J, Scheynius A, Acevedo N, Reinius L, Taub MA, Montano C, Aryee MJ, Feinberg JI, Feinberg AP, Tegnér J, Klareskog L, Catrina AI, Ekström TJ. High-specificity bioinformatics framework for epigenomic profiling of discordant twins reveals specific and shared markers for ACPA and ACPA-positive rheumatoid arthritis. Genome Med. 2016;8(1):124.
[19] Glossop JR, Nixon NB, Emes RD, Sim J, Packham JC, Mattey DL, Farrell WE, Fryer AA. DNA methylation at diagnosis is associated with response to disease-modifying drugs in early rheumatoid arthritis. Epigenomics. 2016, Nov 25. [Epub ahead of print] PMID:27885849.
[20] Scher JU, Sczesnak A, Longman RS, Segata N, Ubeda C, Bielski C, Rostron T, Cerundolo V, Pamer EG, Abramson SB, Huttenhower C, Littman DR. Expansion of intestinal Prevotella copri correlates with enhanced susceptibility to arthritis. Elife. 2013;2:e01202.
[21] Zhang X, Zhang D, Jia H, Feng Q, Wang D, Liang D, Wu X, Li J, Tang L, Li Y, Lan Z, Chen B, Li Y, Zhong H, Xie H, Jie Z, Chen W, Tang S, Xu X, Wang X, Cai X, Liu S, Xia Y, Li J, Qiao X, Al-Aama JY, Chen H, Wang L, Wu QJ, Zhang F, Zheng W, Li Y, Zhang M, Luo G, Xue W, Xiao L, Li J, Chen W, Xu X, Yin Y, Yang H, Wang J, Kristiansen K, Liu L, Li T, Huang Q, Li Y, Wang J. The oral and gut microbiomes are perturbed in rheumatoid arthritis and partly normalized after treatment. Nat Med. 2015;21(8):895-905.
[22] Liu X, Zeng B, Zhang J, Li W, Mou F, Wang H, Zou Q, Zhong B, Wu L, Wei H, Fang Y. Role of the Gut Microbiome in Modulating Arthritis Progression in Mice. Sci Rep. 2016;6:30594.
[23] Gomez A, Luckey D, Yeoman CJ, Marietta EV, Berg Miller ME, Murray JA, White BA, Taneja V. Loss of sex and age driven differences in the gut microbiome characterize arthritis-susceptible 0401 mice but not arthritis-resistant 0402 mice. PLoS One. 2012;7(4):e36095.
[24] Taneja V. Arthritis susceptibility and the gut microbiome. FEBS Lett. 2014;588(22):4244-9.

Lazaros I. Sakkas, MD, DM, PhD(UK), FRCP(UK)
Professor and Chairman
Department of Rheumatology and Clinical Immunology,
Faculty of Medicine, School of Health Sciences,
University of Thessaly, Larissa, Greece

Section 1

Epigenetics in Rheumatoid Arthritis

Chapter 1

MicroRNAs in Rheumatoid Arthritis: From Pathogenesis to Clinical Utility

Agnieszka Paradowska-Gorycka and
Barbara Stypińska

Additional information is available at the end of the chapter

http://dx.doi.org/10.5772/67320

Abstract

Emerging evidence suggests that microRNAs (miRNAs) play a key role in the regulation of immunological functions including innate and adaptive immune responses, development and differentiation of immune cells, and the prevention of autoimmunity. The current state of our knowledge in this area is far from being complete, and continued investigations will be needed to reveal a better understanding of the miRNA network that is involved in the pathogenesis of rheumatoid arthritis (RA). In RA, miRNA plays an important role in many different cellular processes. It has been shown that they modulate inflammatory responses, proliferation of synoviocytes, and production of metalloproteinases in rheumatoid joins and affect the development, differentiation, effector, and regulatory functions of T and B cells and cytokine production. The specific circulating miRNA species may also be useful for the diagnosis, classification, and prognosis of diseases and prediction of the therapeutic response.

Keywords: pathogenesis, epigenetics, microRNA, function of miRNAs, polymorphisms

1. Introduction

Rheumatoid arthritis (RA) is an autoimmune, polygenic disease, which affects millions of people worldwide [1]. Human genetic and epigenetic studies have shown that causal factors of disease include contributions from at least 40 different genes and the effect of environmental factors. Epigenetics represents a new aspect in autoimmunity, which regulates gene expression without alternating DNA sequence. The epigenetic mechanisms are implicated in the final interpretation of the encoded genetic information by regulating gene expression, and alterations in their profile influence the activity of the immune system. Although there are controversies regarding the involvement of genetic and epigenetic factors in RA etiology, it is becoming obvious that the two systems (genetic and epigenetic) interact with each other and are ultimately responsible for RA development.

Recently, the list of molecules important for RA pathogenesis has been extended to microRNAs (miRNAs), which play a central role in regulating both adaptive and innate immune response, development and differentiation of immune cells, and the prevention of autoimmunity [2]. miRNAs regulate protein expression at the posttranscriptional level through reduction of mRNA stability and inhibition of translation [3]. Human miRNA genes are located on all chromosomes except the chromosome Y, are mainly observed in introns (70%), constitute only 3% of the human genome, and regulate about 90% of different genes [4, 5]. These molecules participate in the regulation of the expression of genes involved in the fundamental biological processes related to development, proliferation, and apoptosis, as well as pathological processes including autoimmunity [6, 7].

Although we are still at a very early stage in understanding their impact on immunity, miRNAs are changing the way we think about the development of the immune system and regulation of immune functions. While characterization of miRNA expression patterns in RA patients can have potential diagnostic use, new discoveries in cell type-specific miRNA expression profile, during the disease progression, may provide further understanding of RA pathogenesis. Because miRNAs are stable in plasma or serum, they may be use as biomarkers for the prediction of the disease activity, the differentiation of RA from other rheumatic diseases, or the monitoring of current therapy.

2. Biogenesis

Mature miRNAs are single-stranded, small, noncoding RNAs about 22 nt long. The biogenesis of miRNAs is under tight temporal and spatial control. It starts in nucleus where long primary miRNAs (pri-miRNAs) are transcribed by RNA polymerase II. miRNA sequences are located within various genomic contexts including both intronic and exonic regions. Pri-miRNA transcription is regulated by transcription factors like p53, MYC, ZEB1, ZEB2, and myoblast determination protein 1 (MYOD1). Additionally, epigenetic factors (DNA methylation and histone modifications) regulate this process. The resulting transcript is capped with a specially modified nucleotide at the 5' end (MGpppG) and polyadenylated with a poly(A) tail at 3' end. Pri-miRNA is subsequently cleaved by the so-called microprocessor complex and forms a precursor hairpin miRNA (pre-miRNA). Microprocessor complex is composed of RNase III enzyme—Drosha and of the RNA-binding protein DGCR8 (also known as Pasha). In the next step, pre-miRNA is exported from the nucleus to the cytoplasm in a process involving exportin-5 (Exp-5) and GTP-binding nuclear protein RAN•GTP. Following translocation to the cytoplasm, the pre-miRNA is cleaved, by the cytoplasmic RNase III enzyme Dicer, into 19- to 23-nucleotide mature miRNA duplexes. Although either strand of the duplex may potentially act as a functional miRNA, only one is usually loaded into the RNA-induced silencing complex (RISC) where the miRNA and its mRNA target interact (reviewed by Ref. [8]). miRNA

http://dx.doi.org/10.5772/67320

guides RISC complex to the 3'-untranslated region (3'-UTR) of target mRNA to prevent translation of the mRNA into protein. The other (termed the passenger) strand is degraded or released from the cell. There are few different mechanisms of miRNA export from the cell. miRNAs may be released from the cell by exosomes or microvesicles. Moreover, miRNAs can form complexes with high-density lipoproteins or RNA-binding proteins such as Ago2 and in that form circulate outside the cell. Exact mechanism of how these complexes are transported from the cell still remains unknown. They may be released passively, after cell death, or actively through specific membrane channels or proteins. Interestingly, other pathways for miRNA biogenesis are also emerging. Examples include those that are independent of Drosha or Dicer, "mirtrons"—some small nucleolar RNAs (snoRNAs) and endogenous short hairpin RNAs (shRNAs) [8–10].

3. Mechanism of action

Small noncoding miRNA has the potential to broadly influence various molecular pathways via suppression of unwanted mRNA transcripts. These highly conserved ~22-nucleotide long miRNAs recognize its mRNA target through "seed region" that is located at the 5' end of miRNA and span from nucleotide positions 2–7. It binds to mRNAs' complementary sequence usually located within 3'-untranslated region (3'-UTR). miRNAs silence its target expression via various mechanisms leading to mRNA degradation or preventing mRNA from being translated [11]. After specific mRNA sequence recognition, argonaute (AGO) protein recruits factors that induce translational repression or mRNA degradation. Target mRNA destination depends probably on the sequence complementarity level with miRNA—complete complementarity leads to mRNA degradation and partial complementarity to translational inhibition, although there are exceptions to this rule. Interestingly, some target mRNAs can be exclusively repressed by degradation or translational inhibition, but often it occurs by combination of these two processes (reviewed in Refs. [9, 12]).

3.1. Inhibition of translation

There are still many unknowns around mechanism of translational repression of target mRNA. It is not clear whether miRNA represses translation at the step of translational initiation or posttranslational level [13]. Significant number of studies support model of repression at posttranslational level (protein degradation) or at late stage of translation (premature termination or impaired elongation). These studies demonstrated that miRNA-repressed mRNAs maintained the same distribution pattern across polyribosomes compared with non-repressed mRNAs [14, 15]. However, other studies showed contradictory results, indicating that repression occurs at the translational initiation step. There are many models proposing mechanism of this process.

Almost all proposed models consider GW182 interaction with one of the Ago proteins as a first step of translational repression. In first model, GW182 disrupts the association between eIF4G and poly-A-binding protein (PABP) and prevents the circularization required for efficient translation. In the second model, formation of the mRNA 40S preinitiation complex occurs, but miRISC complex prevents 60S ribosome from joining it, resulting in translation repression. The third scenario assumes that ribosome is detached earlier leading to premature translation termination. Another possible proposed mechanism assumes that target mRNA is accumulated in so-called processing bodies (P-bodies) that prevents from interaction with translational machinery [12, 16].

3.2. Destabilization of target mRNA

There are two mechanisms of miRNA-mediated mRNA degradation-specific cleavage and non-cleavage mRNA degradation. mRNA degradation by miRNA requires Ago, GW182, and the cellular decapping and deadenylation machinery. miRNA sufficient complementarity to target mRNA leads to its specific cleavage. The process is facilitated through Ago protein slicer activity. Ago cleavage site is determined by miRNA sequence, not mRNA paring residues, and occurs within mRNA pairing site to the 10th and 11th residues of miRNA. Therefore, the degree of complementarity at the 3' end of miRNA is more important than at the 5' end. After cleavage miRNA remains intact and is able to mediate another mRNA silencing [17, 18]. Non-cleavage degradation of target mRNA involves GW182. GW182 forms a bridge between RISC and CCR4-NOT deadenylase complex leading to mRNA deadenylation and decapping [19, 20].

4. Biological function of microRNAs

MicroRNAs as endogenous regulatory molecules are present in plant, animal, and human cells, and they are essential for proper development and functioning of the organism. Their main role is associated with posttranscriptional regulation of the expression of numerous genes in both pathogenic and pathological aspects of diseases (**Figure 1**) [21, 22]. miRNAs together with Argonaute (AGO) proteins, forming a core of the miRNA-induced silencing complex (miRISC) which mediates gene silencing [23]. Each miRNA has several different targets, and many of mRNAs are subject to regulation by more than one miRNA [24]. Over 60% of human genes are controlled by miRNAs, which indicates the great importance of these molecules [23].

The continuous miRNA-mRNA interaction is essential for miRNA function. miRNA genes are present either as independent transcription units or located in introns and exons of other genes. Gene silencing can be done either through degradation of a specific mRNA or as a result of the inhibiting of the transcript translation. Furthermore, the mechanisms by which miRNA complementarity to its target mediates repression are varied [25, 26]. In some cases the miRNA binds with complementarity in the seed region (nucleotides 2–8 of the miRNA) within the 3'-untranslated region (UTR) of mRNA and leads to inhibit target gene translation or less commonly within the 5'-UTR region that enhancement of translation [25, 27]. But on the other hand, the miRNA-mRNA interaction occurs in the central region (bases ~9 to 12)

http://dx.doi.org/10.5772/67320

leading to the mRNA cleavage and subsequent degradation [26]. Generally, miRNAs do not act to completely silence their targets, but rather decrease expression. However, the identification of the type of interaction between miRNA and mRNA remains a very important focus to understand control in gene expression [26, 27].

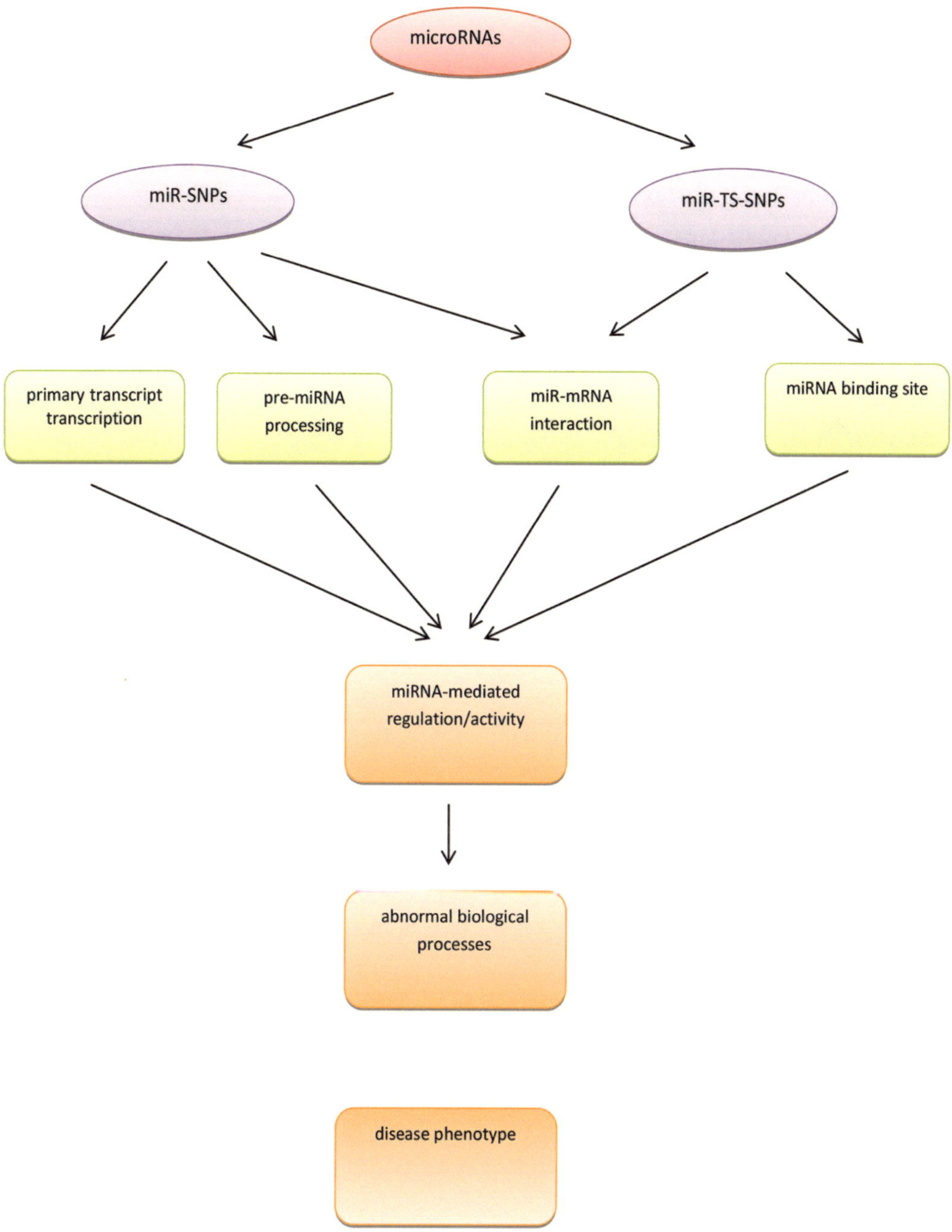

Figure 1. Biological functions of microRNAs.

In the last years, a large number of studies examined cellular miRNA profiles, where expression changes under stress conditions, in cancer, and in other diseases. Distortion of miRNA expression may result in abnormalities in the course of numerous cellular processes, such as development, differentiation, proliferation, inflammation, cell fate determination, apoptosis, signal transduction, organ development, hematopoietic lineage differentiation, host-viral interactions, osteogenesis, and stem cell and germ line proliferation [22, 24, 25, 27–30]. These discoveries may help to clarify molecular mechanisms of diseases and based on this knowledge and may help to develop new drugs. However, since the amount of miRNA may be differ, its total quantity in the different type of cells and gene silencing efficiency depends on the concentration of mRNA targets interpretation of miRNA expression, as well as profiles, including clinical studies, should be performed with attention.

While the majority of miRNAs are found intracellularly, miRNAs may also function beyond RISC, as an extracellular, in virtually all known body fluids [31, 32]. The extracellular miRNAs are secreted into exosomes or microvesicles [26]. However, little is known about the origin of body fluid miRNAs in both healthy and disease conditions or what factors affect their levels in serum/plasma [31]. One hypothesis suggests that blood cells are the major contributors to extracellular miRNAs in the serum or plasma, but another hypothesis speculates that organs may also contribute to extracellular miRNAs because tissue-enriched miRNAs (e.g., miR-122 in the liver, miR-133 in the muscle, miR-208 in the heart, and miR-124 in the brain) are also detected in serum or plasma [31]. Independently of existing hypotheses, explanation of the origin of the extracellular miRNA would increase our understanding of their potential pathophysiological significance. In addition, regardless of their origin, extracellular miRNAs are extremely stable, and their concentration did not significantly change with prolonged incubation of blood plasma at room temperature [23]. The level and composition of extracellular miRNAs in body fluids, such as serum or plasma, are correlated with several pathological conditions, including cancer, diabetes, inflammatory diseases, as well as tissue injury [31]. Moreover, expression patterns of miRNAs are also different between disease state and normal tissue [26] and appear to be tissue specific [21]. However, current knowledge about the biological function of extracellular miRNAs is in its infancy stage. Nevertheless, it seems that extracellular miRNAs may act as signaling molecules and mediate distant cell-cell communication. Cross talk mediated by these miRNAs may provide new insights into the understanding of the mechanisms underlying various dysfunctional conditions. Cross talk through these miRNAs may provide new look at the understanding of the mechanisms underlying the various dysfunctional states [31].

5. Rheumatoid arthritis as a chronic civilization disease

Rheumatoid arthritis is one of the most prevalent chronic inflammatory diseases and is characterized by progressive joint inflammation, by destruction of articular cartilage and underlying bone, and by synovial hyperplasia. RA can affect any joint, with a joint cavity lined by synovial membrane (SM) [33, 34]. The disease process is highly variable, with periods of exacerbation and remission, and uncontrolled inflammation leads to progressive joint damage, pain, long-term disability, and reduced quality of life in many patients [34, 35].

http://dx.doi.org/10.5772/67320

Although RA affects people all over the world, women are affected three times more than men with the peak of incidence between 35 and 55 years of age [33, 36–38]. The incidence of rheumatoid arthritis is relatively constant in most European and North-American populations and is estimate between 0.5% and 1%. RA incidence decreases from north to south and from urban to rural areas. A positive family history increased the risk of RA, and we can see that the familial RA occurrences are about 10–30% of patients, whereas the concordance rate is 12–15% in monozygotic twins and 3–4% in dizygotic twins [39].

RA is pathologically heterogeneous and it is classified among systemic autoimmune disorders because of the presence of rheumatoid factor (RF) and other autoantibodies such as anticitrullinated protein autoantibodies (ACPAs) [35, 40, 41]. RF is present in about 60–85% patients with RA; ACPAs appear to be equally sensitive (75%) and highly specific: 94% for the established disease and 61% for early RA, which may be able to serve as an early diagnostic marker and prognostic factor of joint destruction [42].

Although the exact etiology remains an active area of worldwide research, it is generally accepted that the RA is a multifactorial disease of which pathogenesis is defined by genetic and environmental factors [21]. Genetic predisposition is responsible for 50–60% of the risk of developing RA [43, 44]. A genetic link to RA was established through the observation of familial clustering of RA and large-scale genome-wide association studies (GWAS) [45]. Moreover, it is suggested that only the specific combination of genetic factors in an individual might determine the outcome of the disease [7]. HLA-DRB1 alleles, which share a common sequence, known as the "shared epitope" account for approximately 30% to 50% of overall genetic susceptibility to RA. Probably some other genes associated with components of the innate and adaptive immune system and other mechanisms such as epigenetics may also play a role in the pathogenesis of RA. Epigenetic mechanisms are engaged in the final interpretation of the genetic information by regulation of the gene expression, and changes in their profile influence the activity of the immune system [46]. The change in epigenetic mechanisms is implicated in the final interpretation of the encoded genetic information by regulating gene expression; on the other hand, genetic mutations in epigenetic regulators may alter the epigenetic profile. Consequently, epigenetics and genetics can be two sides of the same coin, as has been determined in the field of rheumatoid arthritis research [46]. Future challenges are understanding and leveraging of the role of genetics and epigenetic modifications, as well as their functional characteristics in RA pathogenesis and translation of fundamental discoveries into clinical practice [47].

6. miRNAs in the pathogenesis of rheumatoid arthritis

Up to date about 2,500 different miRNAs were discovered in humans. From all of these miRNAs, some may play an important role in the regulation of the innate and adaptive immune responses in patients with RA. Increasing number of studies has shown that abnormal miRNA expression in different fluids or cells from RA patients may lead to inflammation, cytokine signaling, bone degradation, and invasive behavior of resident cells [6]. In addition, there is growing evidence that miRNAs as crucial mediators of inflammation may also regulate the plasticity and the effector functions of differentiated Th-cell subsets [24, 48]. miRNAs on the one hand have an important role in defining and maintaining the gene expression programmer of differentiated Th17 cells, but on the other hand, the miRNA expression in regulatory T cells (Treg cells) is important for the maintenance of self-tolerance. And as we know, abnormally activated inflammatory Th cells and defective Treg cells play primary role in the pathogenesis of RA. Moreover, miRNA expression may be also diverse in the different stages of RA progression, allowing miRNAs to help monitor disease activity and help to understand its pathogenesis [6]. Understanding the potential link between miRNAs and the pathogenesis of RA may lead to future insights into disease diagnosis and treatment [4, 22].

The first evidence that miRNAs may be involved in the molecular mechanisms of RA arose in 2007 with the recognition, in the serum of RA patients, of autoantibodies directed against GW bodies that are cytoplasmic structures for storage and/or degradation of mRNA [4]. The first miRNAs that shown abnormal expression within the inflamed joints of RA patients includes miR-16, miR-146a, and miR-155 [4, 49]. These multifunctional miRNAs play a central role in the inflammatory response and immune dysfunction, in response to microbial components, and are upregulated after immune cell maturation [4]. miR-16 and miR-146a play a role in the regulation of the tumor necrosis factor alpha (TNF-α) signaling, which is one of the key cytokines involved on the pathogenesis of RA [2, 50]. Furthermore, miR-155 could suppress matrix metalloproteinases (MMPs) through the interaction with proinflammatory cytokines and Toll-like receptor (TLR) ligands and lead to modulation of joint inflammation [2, 51]. miR-146a and miR-155 are responsible for the maintenance of immune homeostasis, and their expression changes in RA may alert cytokine secretion from different immune cells [30]. Moreover, "miR-146a and miR-155 are considered the 'yin and yang' of inflammation as these miRNAs are negative and positive regulators of inflammatory responses, respectively" [30]. miR-155 promotes T-cell–mediated tissue inflammation by the regulation of the Th1- and Th17-cell response, and it also through the targeting of SOCS1, a negative regulator of IL-2 signaling, controls Treg cell homeostasis [24]. Like miR-155, miR-146a is highly expressed in Treg cells. Furthermore, in contrast to miR-155, miR-146a required for the suppressive activity of Treg cells is essential for the ability of Treg cells to restrain IFN-γ-mediated pathogenic Th1 responses and associated inflammation [24, 50]. Whereas miR-146a rather reduces the proinflammatory immune responses, miR-155 enhances inflammatory processes [48]. The main advantage of the detection of miR-16 and miR-146a in serum/plasma is that this opens the possibility to test as a biomarker to monitoring disease activity/course, because both have shown positive correlation with C-reactive protein (CRP) and disease activity score in 28 joints (DAS28) [4, 48].

Other tissue and/or extracellular miRNAs have been also shown to be associated with RA (**Table 1**), and those miRNAs can regulate specific cytokine pathways, thus leading to inflammation [27]. Characteristics of miRNA profile in patients with RA suggest putative functions of these factors in cytokine secretion and signaling during chronic inflammatory processes in the joints. The miR-10a, miR-16, miR-23b, and miR-203 may serve to fine-tune cytokine signaling, and they may be responsible for the induction of autoimmune inflammation [24, 50]. Upregulation of miR-16 and miR-203 in synovium of RA patients is responsible for the regulation of the TNF-α signaling and for increased matrix metalloproteinases (MMPs), as well as

IL-6 production, respectively, thus indicating that these miRNAs may plays a role as proinflammatory and joint destructive factors [27, 50]. In contrast, miR-10a and miR-23b, which are downregulated in RA synovial tissue, regulate signaling pathway of proinflammatory cytokines such as IL-1β, TNF-α and IL-6, IL-8, and IL-17, as well as MCP-1 and MMPs, and they may be a strong pathological factors that play a critical role in the onset and progression of RA [50, 52]. The cytokines are also a key regulator of Th17/Treg imbalance, which participate in the immune dysfunction. The immune dysfunction in RA patients is found to be induced by decreased expression of miR-21, which may suppress Treg development while promoting Th17 differentiation. Moreover, this miRNA may serve as a novel regulator of Th17/Treg balance in autoimmune diseases including RA [53]. Another miRNA, which participate in the balance between Th17 and Treg cells, is miR-10a, which exhibits high expression in natural Treg cells, limiting the conversion of inducible Treg cells into follicular helper T cells (Tfh cells) and inhibiting Th17 differentiation [54].

miRNAs	Localization	Target gene	Changes	Function
miR-10a	PBMCs, DCs, nTreg cells	STAT - Signal transducer and activator of transcription Foxp3, Bcl-6, Ncor2	Downregulation	- Control IL-6 and IL-21 signaling - Regulate the stability of Treg cells - Limit the conversion of iTreg cells into Tfh cells - Inhibit Th17 differentiation
miR-16	PBMCs, plasma, synovial fluid	TNF-α	Upregulation	- Marker of disease activity
miR-17-92	RASFs, FLS, B cells	MMP-1, IL-6, IL-8, MCP-1, RANTES	Downregulation	- Modulate apoptosis, proliferation - Joint inflammation and destruction - Regulated proinflammatory cytokine production
miR-21	plasma, PBMCs, $CD4^{+}T$	Foxp3 STAT3	Upregulation	- Regulate th17/Treg balance
miR-22	RASFs	CYR61	Downregulation	- Synovial tissue hyperplasia - Th17 differentiation
miR-23b	ST	IL-1β TNF-α IL-17	Downregulation	- Induction of autoimmune inflammation
miR-24	plasma	TGF - transforming growth factor-β1	Upregulation	- Marker of disease activity - Enhance the inflammation
miR-26a	PBMCs, plasma		Upregulation	- Diagnostic biomarker
miR-30a	ST	BECN1 - beclin 1	Downregulation	- Reduce apoptosis

miRNAs	Localization	Target gene	Changes	Function
miR-34a	RASFs	XIAP	Downregulation	- Contribute to apoptosis
miR-124a	RASFs, synoviocytes	CDK-2 MCP-1 VEGF	Downregulation	- Regulator of RASFs and autoimmune inflammation - Contribute to angiogenesis
miR-125b	serum, blood	NF-κB	Downregulation	- Induce of excessive inflammation
miR-146	SF, ST, RASFs, PBMCs, blood, serum, T cells, B cells, monocytes, macrophages	TLR4, NOX4 - NADPH oxidase 4,	Upregulation	- Marker of disease activity - Inhibit Th1-mediated responses - Suppress activity of Treg cells - Modulated apoptosis
miR-155	ST, SF, RASFs, PBMCs, blood, serum, macrophages	SHIP-1, SOCS-1MyD88, MAP3K10 - Mitogen-Activated Protein Kinase Kinase Kinase 10	Upregulation	- Regulate cytokine expression - Require for homeostasis and function of Treg cells
miR-203	RASFs	MMP-1, NF-κB	Upregulation	- Participate in joint inflammatory state
miR-223	PBMCs, RASFs, ST, plasma, macrophages, monocytes, T cells		Upregulation	- Regulate osteoclastogenesis
miR-451	T cells, neutrophils	p38 MAPK - mitogen-activated protein kinases, CPNE3 - copine 3	Downregulation	- Role in inflammation

PBMCs, peripheral blood mononuclear cells; RASFs, RA synovial fibroblasts; FLS, fibroblast-like synoviocytes; MMP-1, matrix metalloproteinase-1; MCP-1, monocyte chemoattractant protein-1; RANTES, regulated on activation, normal T cell expressed and secreted; ST, synovial tissue; XIAP, X-linked inhibitor of apoptosis protein; CDK-2, cyclin-dependent kinase 2; VEGF, vascular endothelial growth factor; SF, synovial fluid; SHIP-1, Src homology 2-containing inositol phosphatase-1

Table 1. Candidate miRNAs for the RA pathogenesis.

Several of different cells, such as T cells, B cells, or macrophages, have been identified as the sources leading to local joint deformation [55]. These cells are the sources of some miRNAs that, through the regulation of the osteoclastogenesis and differentiation of articular chondrocytes, are implicated in the renewal of cartilage and bone degradation [50]. The best known miRNAs involved in joint destruction are miR-146a and miR-155. However, recently marked expression of other miRNAs, miR-223 and miR-19a/b, have been shown within inflamed joint in patients with RA [3, 4, 51, 56]. miR-223 overexpression suppressed the production of osteoclasts and expression of osteoclast-marked genes [50]. Moreover, an inverse correlation between the plasma miR-223 levels and the tender join count was observed [4]. The expression of the miR-19 was downregulated in RA fibroblast-like synoviocytes (FLS), and this plays a role in joint destruction, in response to TLR stimulation [57]. miR-19a and miR-19b negatively regulate the synthesis of IL-6 and regulate the expression of MMP3, suggesting a role of both these miRNAs in protecting patients with RA from joint inflammation and consequently destruction [57].

The above-addressed miRNAs are not only important positive/negative regulators of inflammatory response and immune dysfunction, but they also may be useful for the prediction of the disease course and identification of early pathological events, as well as beneficial for the development of new therapeutic strategies [50].

7. Therapeutic potential of miRNA in treatment of rheumatoid arthritis

The discovery of the miRNA as regulators of gene expression was followed by a wave of interest and intensive studies for elucidating their role both in physiological and pathological conditions. The obtained results raised hopes for the possibility of developing a number of therapeutic uses of these molecules. miRNAs are characterized by many features that make them excellent candidates for biomarker drug entity. These molecules are small with sequence well-known and often conserved among species, which are very attractive features from a drug development standpoint.

Some alterations of miRNA expression have been associated with many human disorders including autoimmune diseases, metabolic disorders, and genetic diseases. By targeting cells affected with improper miRNA expression, the normal balance of the expression can be restored. Novel systems to achieve targeted modulation of specific miRNA in vivo were developed. By controlling the miRNA that regulate mRNAs in cells, they can be used for therapeutic treatment for certain cellular disorders. Individual miRNAs can be targeted using specifically modified antisense oligonucleotides—anti-miRNAs. By virtue of specific modifications, anti-miRNAs gain improved binding affinity, nuclease resistance, and in vivo delivery. For example, 2′-O-methoxyethyl phosphorothioate (MOE) or N,N-diethyl-4-(4-nitronaphthalen-1-ylazo)-phenylamine (ZEN) oligonucleotide modifications were generated to improve binding affinity and block exonuclease degradation. Other examples are anti-miRNAs conjugated to cholesterol to improve its uptake into the cell through the membrane. Furthermore, the great potential seems to lie in the ability of individual miRNAs to regulate the expression of many related genes, which could lead to the regulation of whole signaling pathways or metabolic modulation using one or more miRNA molecules. On the other hand, effect on multiple targets also involves high risk due to the unexpected side effects. Nevertheless, important role of microRNA in regulation of all cellular processes and constant tissue-specific expression indicates its high potential for diagnostic and therapeutic usage [9]. Moreover, miRNA properties and characteristics indicate their excellent potential to be clinical biomarkers. It is well-known that perfect biomarker should be stable in a sample, easy to assess, specific, and sensitive to relevant changes, and miRNA fulfil these criteria. Although cell endogenous miRNA is not very stable and easily degraded, it was discovered that miRNA detected in the blood [21] (plasma, platelets, nucleated blood cells) and synovial fluid [32] is stable and in the case of miRNA in the blood even resistant to harsh condition like high temperature, high and low pH, or multiple freeze-thaw cycles. miRNAs require this surprising stability due to microparticles (exosomes, microvesicles, and apoptotic bodies), RNA-binding proteins (like Ago2), or lipoprotein complexes [high-density lipoprotein (HDL)] that protect them from degradation. The value of miRNA as molecular biomarkers for diagnosis, prognosis, and prediction of therapeutic response is widely documented in cancer. Another advantage that raises interest in the use of circulating miRNAs as clinical biomarkers is fact that there are highly sensitive and specific miRNA detection methods in a quantitative manner, such as real-time PCR, sequencing, and microarrays. In that respect, circulating miRNAs offer many features to make them an attractive class of biomarkers [10].

7.1. miRNA as potential therapeutic agent for RA treatment

The involvement in the pathophysiology of RA coupled with specific characteristics of miRNAs has triggered the scientific community to start exploring the possibilities of viewing miRNAs as therapeutic entities. Especially the potential of a single miRNA to modulate several genes and affect multiple distinct disease-regulatory pathways simultaneously makes miRNAs particularly attractive candidate targets for chronic inflammatory disease as RA. However, only a limited number of groups have explored the therapeutic potential of miRNAs in RA.

Among many approaches considering belief that one miRNA is able to control several genes and pathways, targeting miR-155 represents the most encouraging miRNA-based therapeutic strategy today.

Currently available data clearly show that miR-155 is crucial for the development of arthritis by increasing production of proinflammatory cytokines and promoting differentiation of antigen-specific T cells and antigen-specific antibodies. Interestingly Kurowska-Stolarska et al. observed that miR-155 deficiency is protective against development of collagen-induced arthritis (CIA) in mice. Inhibition of miR155 was associated with impaired production of proinflammatory cytokines, development of the autoreactive Th17 cells, production of anti-collagen II antibodies, and lack of articular inflammation. MiR-155-deficient mice display reductions in both joint inflammation and bone erosion [58]. Beside miR-155, several miRNAs have been implicated in diseases that affect cartilage or have been identified as essential in cartilage homeostasis or repair. For example, the expression of miR-26a was shown to be reduced in splenic cells isolated from rats with induced arthritis. Treatment with methotrexate restored the expression miR-26a to levels comparable to those of non-arthritic controls, and repeated miR-26a injections stabilized disease severity and reduced synovitis, but had no effect on joint destruction [59]. miR-26a can affect bone formation, through angiogenesis and osteogenesis-positive regulation. Overexpression of miR-26a resulted in enhanced bone regeneration coordinated with improved vascularization in mouse, leading to complete repair of the defect [60]. Nakasa et al. demonstrated in vivo and in vitro that miR146a is also able to prevent bone/cartilage destruction. They observed that in $CD14^{+}$ human cells transfected by dsmiR-146a and treated with M-CSF and TNFα or Receptor Activator for Nuclear Factor κ B Ligand (RANKL) for osteoclastogenesis induction—tumor necrosis factor receptor-associated factor 6 (TRAF6) protein levels—and the number of Tartrate-resistant acid phosphatase (TRAP)-positive cells were significantly reduced compared to cells transfected with nonspecific dsRNA. Also osteoclast function was significantly inhibited in those cells. Furthermore they tested the efficacy of ds miR-146a inhibition of bone destruction in vivo and observed that the extent of bone and cartilage destruction was reduced in arthritic mice injected with ds miR-146a compared to mice treated with nonspecific dsRNA. However, despite the inhibition of bone/cartilage destruction by ds miR-146a injection, there was no significant difference in the arthritis score between the ds miR-146a-treated group and the nonspecific dsRNA-treated group suggesting that administration of ds miR-146a alone may not be a sufficient treatment for RA [61]. Another group that observed underexpression of miR-451 in neutrophils isolated from patients with RA used a systemic administration to restore normal expression level of miR-451 in mice with monogenic model of autoimmune arthritis (SKG mice). This approach led to reduction in the number of neutrophils in synovium, by suppressing their migration. This "miR-451" treatment resulted in reduced severity of arthritis in SKG mice suggesting its potential as therapeutic agent in RA [62]. miR-124 was also found to negatively regulate osteoclastogenesis of mouse bone marrow macrophages. In rats with adjuvant-induced arthritis (AIA), miR-124 expression level was significantly decreased. Nakamachi et al. observed that injection of miR-124 into rat AIA joints reduces disease severity. It is probably due to miR-124-mediated targeting of NFATC1, a master transcription factor of osteoclast differentiation. This suggests a potential of miR-124 as future therapeutic entity used for arthritis amelioration [63, 64].

Studies on miRNA-based treatment strategies are rare, but we can expect that these therapies will be developed in the near future. Although mentioned above preclinical studies demonstrate the potential of delivering therapeutic miRNAs, numerous challenges still remain in designing effective and safe delivery of these agents in a cell- or tissue-specific manner. We are still lacking evidence of similar miRNA deregulation in human RA and of the ex vivo correction of disease phenotypes in patient-derived cell or tissue samples. Furthermore, the cellular mechanisms that could explain observed clinical benefits of miRNA therapies still need to be characterized in depth.

7.2. miRNA as RA diagnostic biomarkers

The knowledge about potential value of miRNA as molecular biomarkers for diagnosis, prognosis, and prediction of therapeutic response in RA has been expanded. Several abnormally expressed miRNAs in circulation or inflamed joints in RA have been identified. That suggests theirs potential to be used as biomarkers that help to establish or confirm a diagnosis, monitor the degree of immunologic activity or inflammation, or provide prognostic information regarding disease progression and severity. There are few studies that referred the possibility to use plasma and synovial miRNAs as diagnostic biomarkers that distinguish healthy people from patients with RA or another disease with similar symptoms. For example, upregulation of miR-146a, miR-155, and miR-223 has been shown in various compartments such as serum, blood, synovial fluid, and tissues in patients with RA. Many studies observed elevated levels of expression of miR-146a in different tissues from RA patients; some of them confirm that miR146a level is correlated with disease activity that highlights its significance in RA pathogenesis and diagnostic biomarker potential [51, 65–67]. Elsayed et al. confirmed significant upregulation of miR-146a expression in the whole blood of patients with RA and that miR-146a in diagnostic performance was better than anti-CCP and RF. miR-146a expression level allowed for distinguishing RA patients from healthy controls (HCs) with high sensitivity and specificity (96 and 100%, respectively). Moreover, its expression level was positively correlated with disease activity [68]. It is important to note that these studies are limited by a relatively small number of patients and were conducted in patients from different races and ethnicities. Similarly Kriegsmann et al. observed that miR-146a, miR-155, and miR-223 were significantly elevated in RA compared to osteoarthritis (OA) synovial tissues. The sensitivity and specificity for the detection of RA were 0.76/0.80 for miR-146a, 0.80/0.95 for miR-155, and 0.86/0.81 for miR-223. In combination these miRNAs gave even better results as RA diagnostic biomarker with a sensitivity and specificity of 0.84/0.91, respectively [69]. Murata et al. performed comprehensive array study to find out which miRNAs in plasma samples significantly differentiate patients with RA (patients with high disease activity, who had never received any biological therapy such as the anti-TNF agents) from HCs. They tested eleven preselected candidate miRNAs in 102 patients with RA and 104 HCs and found out that miR-125a-5p, miR-26a, and miR-24 expression levels gave the best results. For miR-24, miR-26a, and miR-125a-5p, the values of sensitivity and the specificity were 63.7 and 89.5%, 53.9 and 94.3%, 64.7 and 89.5%, respectively. These results suggest that plasma miR-24, miR-26a, and miR-125a-5p can be diagnostic biomarkers with high specificity. The combinations of miR-24, miR-30a-5p, and miR-125a-5p (termed ePRAM for "estimated probability of RA by plasma miRNAs") with sensitivity 78.4% and specificity 92.3% are more efficient for RA differentiation and have higher diagnostic significance as biomarkers in RA. These selected miRNAs correlate with disease activity (besides miR-125a-5p) erythrocyte sedymentiation rate (ESR), CRP, RF, ACPA, or DAS28 and not only can be markers for diagnosis of RA but also for disease activity of RA [70]. In a small study, Murata et al. assessed the diagnostic usefulness of plasma miR-132 for patients with RA or OA. They showed that plasma miR-132 differentiate RA and OA patients from healthy controls (83.8% of sensitivity and 80.7% of specificity for RA and 84.0% of sensitivity and 81.2% of specificity for OA) but failed to distinguish them from each other. Interestingly they observed that miRNAs in synovial fluid (miR-16, miR-146a, miR-155, and miR-223) from RA patients were significantly higher than those of patients with OA, suggesting that synovial fluid miRNAs could be a useful tool for diagnosis of RA from OA; however, they did not correlate with clinical variables of RA including DAS28 [32].

Although, evidence that supports the therapeutic potential of miRNA-based strategies is growing, further investigations are required to find suitable miRNAs for utilizing as biomarkers for diagnosis, predicting drug efficacy in order to plan optimal management of RA patients.

7.3. miRNA as response to treatment biomarkers

Almost all newly diagnosed RA patients enter their treatment with methotrexate monotherapy. If it fails (and it is ineffective in 66% of patients), other disease-modifying antirheumatic drugs (DMARD) and then one of biologic agents are prescribed. Considering that each type of biology treatment targets different inflammatory mechanisms, sometimes it may take some time to find the best therapy for a patient. Although biological medicines significantly improved RA treatment, there are still some stumbling blocks to be overcome. The major problems of the treatment with biologics are serious potential side effects and high cost of biologics. Currently clinical and serological markers that sufficient predict disease outcome are unavailable. Therefore one of the most challenging issues is the identification of biomarkers that will predict therapeutic outcome and thus would improve patient care and medical cost-effectiveness. Potential value of miRNAs as molecular biomarker for prognosis treatment response is still unexplored in RA. However, there are several reports demonstrating possibility to use them as therapy outcome predictors [6, 71]. Duroux-Richard and Jorgensen proposed hsa-miR-23a-3p and hsa-miR-223-3p as predictors of therapy response and biomarkers of response to anti-TNFα/DMARDs combination therapy. Strong increase in hsa-miR-23a-3p and hsa-miR-223-3p expressions indicated good response to treatment. Moreover those changes significantly correlated with clinical and inflammatory parameters (such as DAS28, CRP, or ESR). Most importantly expression level of these miRNAs showed its potential to predict therapy outcome. hsa-miR-23-3p and hsa-miR-223-3p levels were predictors of nonresponse to anti–TNF-α/DMARD combination treatment with a sensitivity of 62.5 and 57.1% and a specificity of 86.4 and 90.2%, respectively. The combination of these two miRNAs demonstrated an increase in both the sensitivity (62.5%) and specificity (91.5%) in relation to those given by each miRNA alone [6].

Another circulating miRNAs suggested to be a potential predictive biomarker of response to RA treatment was miR-125b. Duroux-Richard et al. observed that miR-125b expression significantly distinguish RA patients from healthy donors and OA patients but not from patients with other rheumatic disorders like tumor necrosis factor receptor-associated periodic syndrome (TRAPS) or spondyloarthritis (SpA). Results obtained in this study also showed that high expression of miR-125b was associated with good response to rituximab therapy. Serum expression levels of tested miRNA before treatment were significantly higher in good responders than in nonresponders. However, it was not correlated with disease activity parameters. These data suggest miR-125b might be considered as a biomarker that predicts therapy response but is not useful as disease activity marker [72].

The realization of personalized medicine requires comprehensive understanding of genetic and nongenetic factors that may be responsible for drug response. Although several miRNAs appear to be attractive molecular biomarkers, discovery of perfect biomarkers for RA diagnosis and prediction of treatment outcome is still in the future. Better understanding of the role of miRNAs in RA pathogenesis and identification of specific miRNA expression patterns in RA may provide novel molecular prognostic and diagnostic biomarker markers and new gene therapy strategies for treating RA.

8. miRNA polymorphisms

As mentioned, RA is a common, but heterogeneous, disease with the heritability about 60 % [73]. As genetic variants are present at birth, genetic studies can help us identify the key genes and pathways that contribute to both occurrence and severity of disease [74]. The last 60 years provided evidence for the genetic basis of rheumatoid arthritis by identifying genetic susceptibility variants. Three basic approaches were applied to recognize these susceptibility loci: candidate single nucleotide polymorphisms (SNPs), linkage, and genome-wide association studies (GWAS), which genotype thousands to millions of SNPs in large human samples. However, more than 10 years after the completion of the human genome sequencing project and numerous GWA studies, we still do not fully understand the genetic basis of RA [74, 75].

Since miRNAs are an important class of regulators of gene expression, genetic polymorphisms located in miRNA genes (miR-SNPs) and/or in miRNA binding sites of target genes (miR-TS-SNPs) can act as regulatory SNPs through modifying the activity of miRNAs to affect the susceptibility to and/or severity of disease (**Figure 2**) [76, 77]. The miR-SNPs are thought to affect function in one of three ways. First, genetic alternation in miRNA genes affects its expression through the transcription of the primary transcript; second, via altering pri-miRNA and pre-miRNA processing; and third, by affecting the miRNA-mRNA interactions [77–79]. In contrast to SNPs in miRNA genes, the miR-TS-SNPs, which are present at or near a miRNA binding site in 3'-untranslated region (UTR) of the target gene, are abundant in the human genome [80]. These SNPs can potentially alter miRNA function by creating as well as destroying a miRNA binding site [78]. Moreover, the functional impact of miR-TS-SNPs on disease phenotype largely depends on whether the corresponding miRNA is expressed in a particular tissue and the expression of other possibly compensatory miRNAs [77]. Prediction of SNPs that could alter the expression of a miRNA or its complementarily with the target genes, and as a result the normal function of the involved molecular pathway, seems to be of great importance [79]. Moreover, the polymorphisms associated with miRNAs may have a more important role in RA disease onset and progression than originally suspected. However, to date only a limited number of studies have identified miR-SNPs and/or miR-TS-SNPs relevant to RA (**Table 1**) [81, 82]. In a genome-wide interaction analysis, miR-146a and miR-499 have received much attention in this field. Up today, miR-146a, the most studied miRNAs in patients with RA, is encoded by chromosome 5q33 and can bind to the 3'-UTR of many target mRNAs, including interleukin-1 receptor-associated kinase 1 (IRAK-1), tumor necrosis factor receptor-associated factor 6 (TRAF-6), and other transcripts associated with inflammatory signaling [83, 84]. The common miR-146a polymorphism [85, 85], which may affect the stability of the miRNA, thereby influencing its expression level [82, 86], is not associated with susceptibility to RA [81, 85, 87], but the miRNA-146a rs2910164 variant might increase the risk of RA in the female population and may influence disease activity [84]. Moreover, it remains unclear which allele is associated with a significantly higher level of mature miR-146a. On the other hand, miR-499, the gene of which is located on 20q11.22 chromosome, targets IL-17 receptor B (IL-17RB), IL-23a, IL-2 receptor B (IL-2Rβ), IL-6, IL-2, B- and T-lymphocyte attenuator, IL-18 receptor (IL-18R), IL-21, peptidyl arginine deiminase type 4 (PADI4), and regulatory factor X 4 (influences human leukocyte antigen class II expression) [83, 84]. The miR-499 polymorphism at position rs3746444T > C, located within the stem region of the miR-499 gene is closely associated with the inflammation of RA and can serve a potential diagnostic biomarker for RA [81, 84]. To date, very little is known about the role of miRNA SNPs in the pathogenesis of RA, and even less is known about whether it could affect miRNA-mRNA interactions. That way, the mechanism by which sequence variations—due to genetic or posttranscriptional changes—in miRNAs and/or in their target genes that modulate miRNA binding characteristics or miRNA expression can affects the inflammatory processes requires further functional studies. With the development of large-scale RNA-sequencing methods, a new light could be shed on these mechanisms [80].

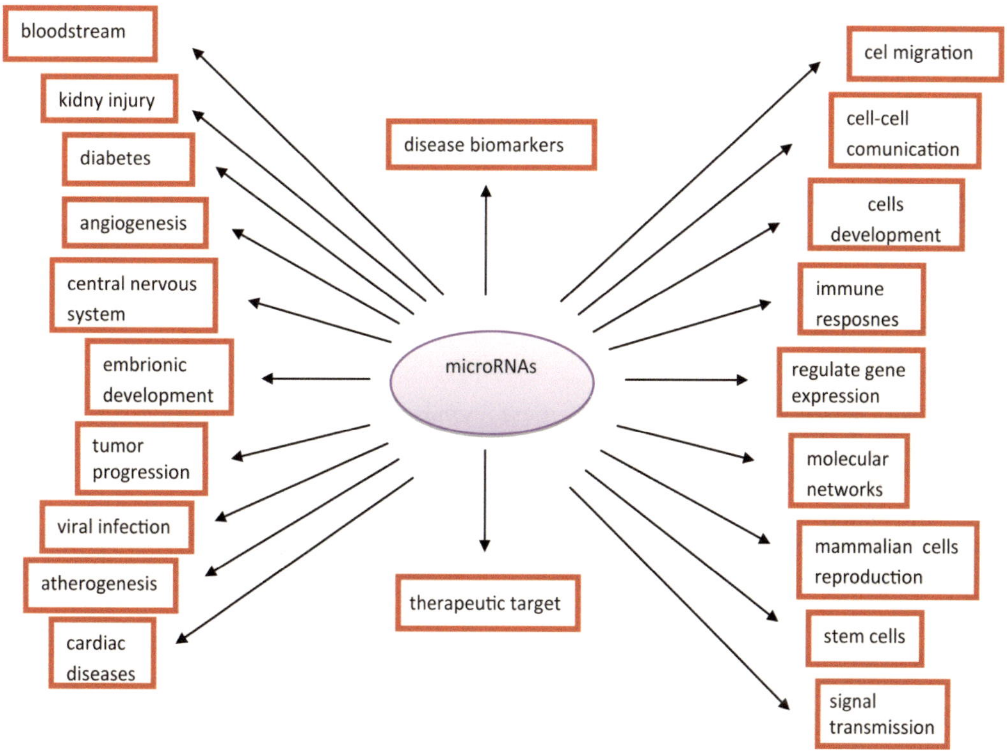

Figure 2. Single nucleotide polymorphisms located in miRNAs.

9. Conclusion

RA is a syndrome in which many different elements of the immune system become activated. A growing number of GWAS demonstrated that genetic polymorphisms, the standard genetic marker to identify associated alleles, make a substantial but incomplete contribution to the risk of RA developing. Now it is widely accepted that epigenetic mechanisms such as miRNAs, a class of powerful and major gene regulators, are also involved in the coordination of the immune processes in the rheumatoid arthritis. Both tissue and extracellular miRNAs are not only key molecules in the molecular mechanisms of the disease but also are very important biomarkers for several pathological conditions and represent a promising therapeutic approach in future. Circulating miRNAs may be suitable for clinical use as they are stable present in body fluids such as plasma or serum. Recent evidence has suggested that miRNA levels in serum or plasma are often higher than in the synovial fluid. In addition, miRNA expression profiles in synovial fluids were similar to those in synovial tissues. These findings demonstrated that synovial tissues and infiltrating cells are the primary source of synovial fluid miRNAs. In contrast, miRNAs that are presented in the serum or plasma are released by several tissues and cells different from those in synovium [32]. Because rheumatoid arthritis is a systemic disease which can have not only a joint involvement but also other organs may be affected, cell-free circulating miRNA signature in serum or plasma is of great interest.

Acknowledgements

This work was supported by a grant from the Polish National Science Center (2015/19/B/NZ5/00247).

Author details

Agnieszka Paradowska-Gorycka* and Barbara Stypińska

*Address all correspondence to: paradowska_aga@interia.pl

Department of Biochemistry and Molecular Biology, National Institute of Geriatrics, Rheumatology and Rehabilitation, Warsaw, Poland

References

[1] Klein K, Gay S. Epigenetic modifications in rheumatoid arthritis, a review. Curr Opin Pharmacol. 2013;13(3):420-425. doi:10.1016/j.coph.2013.01.007.

[2] Salehi E, Eftekhari R, Oraei M, Gharib A, Bidad K. MicroRNAs in rheumatoid arthritis. Clin Rheumatol. 2015;34(4):615-628. doi:10.1007/s10067-015-2898-x.

[3] Filková M, Aradi B, Senolt L, et al. Association of circulating miR-223 and miR-16 with disease activity in patients with early rheumatoid arthritis. Ann Rheum Dis. 2014;73(10):1898-1904. doi:10.1136/annrheumdis-2012-202815.

[4] Duroux-Richard I, Jorgensen C, Apparailly F. What do microRNAs mean for rheumatoid arthritis? Arthritis Rheum. 2012;64(1):11-20. doi:10.1002/art.30651.

[5] Singh RP, Massachi I, Manickavel S, et al. The role of miRNA in inflammation and autoimmunity. Autoimmun Rev. 2013;12(12):1160-1165. doi:10.1016/j.autrev.2013.07.003.

[6] Castro-Villegas C, Pérez-Sánchez C, Escudero A, et al. Circulating miRNAs as potential biomarkers of therapy effectiveness in rheumatoid arthritis patients treated with anti-TNFα. Arthritis Res Ther. 2015;17(1):49. doi:10.1186/s13075-015-0555-z.

[7] Smigielska-Czepiel K, van den Berg A, Jellema P, et al. Comprehensive analysis of miRNA expression in T-cell subsets of rheumatoid arthritis patients reveals defined

signatures of naive and memory Tregs. Genes Immun. 2014;15(2):115-125. doi:10.1038/gene.2013.69.

[8] Ha M, Kim VN. Regulation of microRNA biogenesis. Nat Rev Mol Cell Biol. 2014;15(8):509-524. doi:10.1038/nrm3838.

[9] Bhaskaran M, Mohan M. MicroRNAs: history, biogenesis, and their evolving role in animal development and disease. Vet Pathol. 2014;51(4):759-774. doi:10.1177/0300985813502820.

[10] Creemers EE, Tijsen AJ, Pinto YM. Circulating microRNAs: novel biomarkers and extracellular communicators in cardiovascular disease? Circ Res. 2012;110(3):483-495. doi:10.1161/CIRCRESAHA.111.247452.

[11] Kawano S, Nakamachi Y. The role of miRNA, in Rheumatoid Arthritis. Rheum Arthritis – Etiol Consequences Co-Morbidities. 2012. doi:10.5772/25861.

[12] Gu S, Kay MA, Carthew R, et al. How do miRNAs mediate translational repression? Silence. 2010;1(1):11. doi:10.1186/1758-907X-1-11.

[13] Bartel DP. MicroRNAs: genomics, biogenesis, mechanism, and function. Cell. 2004;116(2):281-297. doi:10.1016/S0092-8674(04)00045-5.

[14] Petersen CP, Bordeleau M-E, Pelletier J, Sharp PA. Short RNAs repress translation after initiation in mammalian cells. Mol Cell. 2006;21(4):533-542. doi:10.1016/j.molcel.2006.01.031.

[15] Nottrott S, Simard MJ, Richter JD. Human let-7a miRNA blocks protein production on actively translating polyribosomes. Nat Struct Mol Biol. 2006;13(12):1108-1114. doi:10.1038/nsmb1173.

[16] Wahid F, Shehzad A, Khan T, Kim YY. MicroRNAs: synthesis, mechanism, function, and recent clinical trials. Biochim Biophys Acta – Mol Cell Res. 2010;1803(11):1231-1243. doi:10.1016/j.bbamcr.2010.06.013.

[17] Hutvágner G, Zamore PD. A microRNA in a multiple-turnover RNAi enzyme complex. Science. 2002;297(5589):2056-2060. doi:10.1126/science.1073827.

[18] Llave C, Xie Z, Kasschau KD, Carrington JC. Cleavage of Scarecrow-like mRNA targets directed by a class of Arabidopsis miRNA. Science. 2002;297(5589):2053-2056. doi:10.1126/science.1076311.

[19] Behm-Ansmant I, Rehwinkel J, Doerks T, Stark A, Bork P, Izaurralde E. mRNA degradation by miRNAs and GW182 requires both CCR4:NOT deadenylase and DCP1:DCP2 decapping complexes. Genes Dev. 2006;20(14):1885-1898. doi:10.1101/gad.1424106.

[20] Wu L, Fan J, Belasco JG. MicroRNAs direct rapid deadenylation of mRNA. Proc Natl Acad Sci U S A. 2006;103(11):4034-4039. doi:10.1073/pnas.0510928103.

[21] Mitchell PS, Parkin RK, Kroh EM, et al. Circulating microRNAs as stable blood-based markers for cancer detection. Proc Natl Acad Sci U S A. 2008;105(30):10513-10518. doi:10.1073/pnas.0804549105.

[22] Huang R-Y, Li L, Wang M-J, Chen X-M, Huang Q-C, Lu C-J. An exploration of the role of microRNAs in psoriasis: a systematic review of the literature. Medicine (Baltimore). 2015;94(45):e2030. doi:10.1097/MD.0000000000002030.

[23] Makarova JA, Shkurnikov MU, Wicklein D, et al. Intracellular and extracellular microRNA: an update on localization and biological role. Prog Histochem Cytochem. 2016;51:33–49. doi:10.1016/j.proghi.2016.06.001.

[24] Baumjohann D, Ansel KM. MicroRNA-mediated regulation of T helper cell differentiation and plasticity. Nat Rev Immunol. 2013;13(9):666-678. doi:10.1038/nri3494.

[25] Miao C-G, Xiong Y-Y, Yu H, et al. Critical roles of microRNAs in the pathogenesis of systemic sclerosis: New advances, challenges and potential directions. Int Immunopharmacol. 2015;28(1):626-633. doi:10.1016/j.intimp.2015.07.042.

[26] Mohr AM, Mott JL. Overview of microRNA biology. Semin Liver Dis. 2015;35(1):3-11. doi:10.1055/s-0034-1397344.

[27] Ceribelli A, Nahid MA, Satoh M, Chan EKL. MicroRNAs in rheumatoid arthritis. FEBS Lett. 2011;585(23):3667-3674. doi:10.1016/j.febslet.2011.05.020.

[28] Huang C, Geng J, Jiang S. MicroRNAs in regulation of osteogenic differentiation of mesenchymal stem cells. Cell Tissue Res. 2016. doi:10.1007/s00441-016-2462-2.

[29] Gao Y, Peng J, Ren Z, et al. Functional regulatory roles of microRNAs in atherosclerosis. Clin Chim Acta. 2016;460:164-171. doi:10.1016/j.cca.2016.06.044.

[30] Vicente R, Noël D, Pers Y-M, Apparailly F, Jorgensen C. Deregulation and therapeutic potential of microRNAs in arthritic diseases. Nat Rev Rheumatol. 2016;12(4):211-220. doi:10.1038/nrrheum.2015.162.

[31] Liang H, Gong F, Zhang S, Zhang C-Y, Zen K, Chen X. The origin, function, and diagnostic potential of extracellular microRNAs in human body fluids. Wiley Interdiscip Rev RNA. 5(2):285-300. doi:10.1002/wrna.1208.

[32] Murata K, Yoshitomi H, Tanida S, et al. Plasma and synovial fluid microRNAs as potential biomarkers of rheumatoid arthritis and osteoarthritis. Arthritis Res Ther. 2010;12(3):R86. doi:10.1186/ar3013.

[33] Tanaka Y. Current concepts in the management of rheumatoid arthritis. Korean J Intern Med. 2016;31(2):210-218. doi:10.3904/kjim.2015.137.

[34] Mimori T. Clinical significance of anti-CCP antibodies in rheumatoid arthritis. Intern Med. 2005;44(11):1122-1126. http://www.ncbi.nlm.nih.gov/pubmed/16357447. Accessed August 25, 2016.

[35] Paradowska A, Maślińiski W, Grzybowska-Kowalczyk A, Łacki J. The function of interleukin 17 in the pathogenesis of rheumatoid arthritis. Arch Immunol Ther Exp (Warsz). 55(5):329-334. http://www.ncbi.nlm.nih.gov/pubmed/18219763. Accessed August 25, 2016.

[36] Kelly M. Robert BRIDGES: pioneer in rheumatology. Med Hist. 1961;5:297-299. http://www.ncbi.nlm.nih.gov/pubmed/13752390. Accessed August 25, 2016.

[37] Cobb S, Kasl S V. The epidemiology of rheumatoid arthritis. Am J Public Health Nations Health. 1966;56(10):1657-1663. http://www.ncbi.nlm.nih.gov/pubmed/5951485. Accessed August 25, 2016.

[38] Williams EA, Fye KH. Rheumatoid arthritis. Targeted interventions can minimize joint destruction. Postgrad Med. 2003;114(5):19-28. http://www.ncbi.nlm.nih.gov/pubmed/14650090. Accessed August 25, 2016.

[39] Reveille JD. Genetic studies in the rheumatic diseases: present status and implications for the future. J Rheumatol Suppl. 2005;72:10-13. http://www.ncbi.nlm.nih.gov/pubmed/15660456. Accessed August 25, 2016.

[40] Romagnani S. Human Th17 cells. Arthritis Res Ther. 2008;10(2):206. doi:10.1186/ar2392.

[41] Layh-Schmitt G, Colbert RA. The interleukin-23/interleukin-17 axis in spondyloarthritis. Curr Opin Rheumatol. 2008;20(4):392-397. doi:10.1097/BOR.0b013e328303204b.

[42] Sakaguchi S, Yamaguchi T, Nomura T, Ono M. Regulatory T cells and immune tolerance. Cell. 2008;133(5):775-787. doi:10.1016/j.cell.2008.05.009.

[43] Awasthi A, Kuchroo VK. Th17 cells: from precursors to players in inflammation and infection. Int Immunol. 2009;21(5):489-498. doi:10.1093/intimm/dxp021.

[44] Bax M, van Heemst J, Huizinga TWJ, Toes REM. Genetics of rheumatoid arthritis: what have we learned? Immunogenetics. 2011;63(8):459-466. doi:10.1007/s00251-011-0528-6.

[45] Viatte S, Plant D, Raychaudhuri S. Genetics and epigenetics of rheumatoid arthritis. Nat Rev Rheumatol. 2013;9(3):141-153. doi:10.1038/nrrheum.2012.237.

[46] Glant TT, Mikecz K, Rauch TA. Epigenetics in the pathogenesis of rheumatoid arthritis. BMC Med. 2014;12:35. doi:10.1186/1741-7015-12-35.

[47] Bottini N, Firestein GS. Epigenetics in rheumatoid arthritis: a primer for rheumatologists. Curr Rheumatol Rep. 2013;15(11):372. doi:10.1007/s11926-013-0372-9.

[48] Zhou Q, Haupt S, Kreuzer JT, et al. Decreased expression of miR-146a and miR-155 contributes to an abnormal Treg phenotype in patients with rheumatoid arthritis. Ann Rheum Dis. 2015;74(6):1265-1274. doi:10.1136/annrheumdis-2013-204377.

[49] Kim T-H, Choi SJ, Lee YH, Song GG, Ji JD. Gene expression profile predicting the response to anti-TNF treatment in patients with rheumatoid arthritis; analysis of GEO datasets. Joint Bone Spine. 2014;81(4):325-330. doi:10.1016/j.jbspin.2014.01.013.

[50] Churov A V, Oleinik EK, Knip M. MicroRNAs in rheumatoid arthritis: altered expression and diagnostic potential. Autoimmun Rev. 2015;14(11):1029-1037. doi:10.1016/j.autrev.2015.07.005.

[51] Stanczyk J, Pedrioli DML, Brentano F, et al. Altered expression of microRNA in synovial fibroblasts and synovial tissue in rheumatoid arthritis. Arthritis Rheum. 2008;58(4):1001-1009. doi:10.1002/art.23386.

[52] Mu N, Gu J, Huang T, et al. A novel NF-κB/YY1/microRNA-10a regulatory circuit in fibroblast-like synoviocytes regulates inflammation in rheumatoid arthritis. Sci Rep. 2016;6:20059. doi:10.1038/srep20059.

[53] Dong L, Wang X, Tan J, et al. Decreased expression of microRNA-21 correlates with the imbalance of Th17 and Treg cells in patients with rheumatoid arthritis. J Cell Mol Med. 2014;18(11):2213-2224. doi:10.1111/jcmm.12353.

[54] Takahashi H, Kanno T, Nakayamada S, et al. TGF-β and retinoic acid induce the microRNA miR-10a, which targets Bcl-6 and constrains the plasticity of helper T cells. Nat Immunol. 2012;13(6):587-595. doi:10.1038/ni.2286.

[55] Chen X-M, Huang Q-C, Yang S-L, et al. Role of microRNAs in the pathogenesis of rheumatoid arthritis: novel perspectives based on review of the literature. Medicine (Baltimore). 2015;94(31):e1326. doi:10.1097/MD.0000000000001326.

[56] Lu M-C, Yu C-L, Chen H-C, Yu H-C, Huang H-B, Lai N-S. Increased miR-223 expression in T cells from patients with rheumatoid arthritis leads to decreased insulin-like growth factor-1-mediated interleukin-10 production. Clin Exp Immunol. 2014;177(3):641-651. doi:10.1111/cei.12374.

[57] Philippe L, Alsaleh G, Suffert G, et al. TLR2 expression is regulated by microRNA miR-19 in rheumatoid fibroblast-like synoviocytes. J Immunol. 2012;188(1):454-461. doi:10.4049/jimmunol.1102348.

[58] Kurowska-Stolarska M, Alivernini S, Ballantine LE, et al. MicroRNA-155 as a proinflammatory regulator in clinical and experimental arthritis. Proc Natl Acad Sci U S A. 2011;108(27):11193-11198. doi:10.1073/pnas.1019536108.

[59] Jiang C, Zhu W, Xu J, et al. MicroRNA-26a negatively regulates toll-like receptor 3 expression of rat macrophages and ameliorates pristane induced arthritis in rats. Arthritis Res Ther. 2014;16(1):R9. doi:10.1186/ar4435.

[60] Li Y, Fan L, Liu S, et al. The promotion of bone regeneration through positive regulation of angiogenic-osteogenic coupling using microRNA-26a. Biomaterials. 2013;34(21):5048-5058. doi:10.1016/j.biomaterials.2013.03.052.

[61] Pauley KM, Cha S. miRNA-146a in rheumatoid arthritis: a new therapeutic strategy. Immunotherapy. 2011;3(7):829-831. doi:10.2217/imt.11.70.

[62] Murata K, Yoshitomi H, Furu M, et al. MicroRNA-451 down-regulates neutrophil chemotaxis via p38 MAPK. Arthritis Rheumatol (Hoboken, NJ). 2014;66(3):549-559. doi:10.1002/art.38269.

[63] Nakamachi Y, Ohnuma K, Uto K, Noguchi Y, Saegusa J, Kawano S. MicroRNA-124 inhibits the progression of adjuvant-induced arthritis in rats. Ann Rheum Dis. 2016;75(3):601-608. doi:10.1136/annrheumdis-2014-206417.

[64] Lee Y, Kim HJ, Park CK, et al. MicroRNA-124 regulates osteoclast differentiation. Bone. 2013;56(2):383-389. doi:10.1016/j.bone.2013.07.007.

[65] Niimoto T, Nakasa T, Ishikawa M, et al. MicroRNA-146a expresses in interleukin-17 producing T cells in rheumatoid arthritis patients. BMC Musculoskelet Disord. 2010;11(1):209. doi:10.1186/1471-2474-11-209.

[66] Pauley KM, Satoh M, Chan AL, Bubb MR, Reeves WH, Chan EK. Upregulated miR-146a expression in peripheral blood mononuclear cells from rheumatoid arthritis patients. Arthritis Res Ther. 2008;10(4):R101. doi:10.1186/ar2493.

[67] Abou-Zeid A, Saad M, Soliman E. MicroRNA 146a expression in rheumatoid arthritis: association with tumor necrosis factor-alpha and disease activity. Genet Test Mol Biomarkers. 2011;15(11):807-812. doi:10.1089/gtmb.2011.0026.

[68] Elsayed HMA, Khater WS, Ibrahim AA, Hamdy MSE, Morshedy NA. MicroRNA-146a expression as a potential biomarker for rheumatoid arthritis in Egypt. Egypt J Med Hum Genet. 2016. doi:10.1016/j.ejmhg.2016.07.001.

[69] Kriegsmann M, Randau TM, Gravius S, et al. Expression of miR-146a, miR-155, and miR-223 in formalin-fixed paraffin-embedded synovial tissues of patients with rheumatoid arthritis and osteoarthritis. Virchows Arch. 2016;469(1):93-100. doi:10.1007/s00428-016-1939-4.

[70] Murata K, Furu M, Yoshitomi H, et al. Comprehensive microRNA analysis identifies miR-24 and miR-125a-5p as plasma biomarkers for rheumatoid arthritis. PLoS One. 2013;8(7):e69118. doi:10.1371/journal.pone.0069118.

[71] Duroux-Richard I, Jorgensen C, Apparailly F. miRNAs and rheumatoid arthritis – promising novel biomarkers. Swiss Med Wkly. 2011. doi:10.4414/smw.2011.13175.

[72] Duroux-Richard I, Pers Y-M, Fabre S, et al. Circulating miRNA-125b is a potential biomarker predicting response to rituximab in rheumatoid arthritis. Mediators Inflamm. 2014;2014:342524. doi:10.1155/2014/342524.

[73] Kurkó J, Besenyei T, Laki J, Glant TT, Mikecz K, Szekanecz Z. Genetics of rheumatoid arthritis – a comprehensive review. Clin Rev Allergy Immunol. 2013;45(2):170-179. doi:10.1007/s12016-012-8346-7.

[74] Raychaudhuri S. Recent advances in the genetics of rheumatoid arthritis. Curr Opin Rheumatol. 2010;22(2):109-118. doi:10.1097/BOR.0b013e328336474d.

[75] Sethupathy P, Collins FS. MicroRNA target site polymorphisms and human disease. Trends Genet. 2008;24(10):489-497. doi:10.1016/j.tig.2008.07.004.

[76] Gong J, Tong Y, Zhang H-M, et al. Genome-wide identification of SNPs in microRNA genes and the SNP effects on microRNA target binding and biogenesis. Hum Mutat. 2012;33(1):254-263. doi:10.1002/humu.21641.

[77] Dole NS, Delany AM. MicroRNA variants as genetic determinants of bone mass. Bone. 2016;84:57-68. doi:10.1016/j.bone.2015.12.016.

[78] Ryan BM, Robles AI, Harris CC. Genetic variation in microRNA networks: the implications for cancer research. Nat Rev Cancer. 2010;10(6):389-402. doi:10.1038/nrc2867.

[79] Jin Y, Lee CGL. Single nucleotide polymorphisms associated with microRNA regulation. Biomolecules. 2013;3(2):287-302. doi:10.3390/biom3020287.

[80] Pivarcsi A, Ståhle M, Sonkoly E. Genetic polymorphisms altering microRNA activity in psoriasis – a key to solve the puzzle of missing heritability? Exp Dermatol. 2014;23(9):620-624. doi:10.1111/exd.12469.

[81] Yang B, Chen J, Li Y, et al. Association of polymorphisms in pre-miRNA with inflammatory biomarkers in rheumatoid arthritis in the Chinese Han population. Hum Immunol. 2012;73(1):101-106. doi:10.1016/j.humimm.2011.10.005.

[82] Chatzikyriakidou A, Voulgari P V, Georgiou I, Drosos AA. miRNAs and related polymorphisms in rheumatoid arthritis susceptibility. Autoimmun Rev. 2012;11(9):636-641. doi:10.1016/j.autrev.2011.11.004.

[83] Xu HY, Wang ZY, Chen JF, et al. Association between ankylosing spondylitis and the miR-146a and miR-499 polymorphisms. PLoS One. 2015;10(4):e0122055. doi:10.1371/journal.pone.0122055.

[84] El-Shal AS, Aly NM, Galil SMA, Moustafa MA, Kandel WA. Association of microRNAs genes polymorphisms with rheumatoid arthritis in Egyptian female patients. Joint Bone Spine. 2013;80(6):626-631. doi:10.1016/j.jbspin.2013.03.005.

[85] Zhou X, Zhu J, Zhang H, Zhou G, Huang Y, Liu R. Is the microRNA-146a (rs2910164) polymorphism associated with rheumatoid arthritis? Association of microRNA-146a (rs2910164) polymorphism and rheumatoid arthritis could depend on gender. Joint Bone Spine. 2015;82(3):166-171. doi:10.1016/j.jbspin.2014.12.009.

[86] Apparailly F. Looking for microRNA polymorphisms as new rheumatoid arthritis risk loci? Joint Bone Spine. 2010;77(5):377-379. doi:10.1016/j.jbspin.2010.06.002.

[87] Li K, Tie H, Hu N, et al. Association of two polymorphisms rs2910164 in miRNA-146a and rs3746444 in miRNA-499 with rheumatoid arthritis: a meta-analysis. Hum Immunol. 2014;75(7):602-608. doi:10.1016/j.humimm.2014.05.002.

Chapter 2

Role of MicroRNAs in Rheumatoid Arthritis

Merih Birlik, Ayşe Koçak and Duygu Harmancı

Additional information is available at the end of the chapter

http://dx.doi.org/10.5772/67081

Abstract

Rheumatoid arthritis (RA) is a common autoimmune disease. The hallmarks of RA are synovial inflammation and hyperplasia, autoantibody production, systemic features, and deformity. A lot of researchers have paid attention to the possibility that microRNAs (miRNAs) play a role in the pathogenesis of RA. miRNAs are a class of small noncoding RNAs, which have 18–25 nucleotides. These small RNAs modify gene expression by binding to target messenger RNA (mRNA), and they block the translation or induce the degradation of target mRNA. Biological relevance of miRNAs has been investigated in physiological and pathological conditions. A growing body of evidence suggests that miRNAs participate in the inflammatory disorders including RA. In this chapter, an overview of biogenesis and function of miRNAs has been presented to introduce researchers to the changes and functional regulation of the key miRNAs in RA and to provide current knowledge in miRNA and RA. It is important to understand the relationship between the key miRNAs and RA pathology as modulation of specific miRNA alterations could be of great pharmaceutical interest in the future.

Keywords: microRNA, miRNA, small noncoding RNA, rheumatoid arthritis, pathogenesis

1. Introduction

Rheumatoid arthritis (RA) is an autoimmune disease characterized by chronic synovial inflammation exemplified by cell hyperplasia, autoantibody production, systemic features, and deformity [1–3]. It affects approximately 0.36–2.0% of the human population worldwide and roughly three to four times more females than males [2, 4]. RA progression is a complex process and consists of many genes and environmental factors [3]. Accumulating clinical and experimental evidence points out that the immune system plays a key role in disease pathogenesis. However, pathogenesis of RA is not entirely clear [1–3]. Generally, RA progression leads to joint destruction, functional disability, and cardiovascular comorbidities [5]. The immune system and different cell types such as macrophages, T and B cells, and synovial fibroblasts participate in the pathogenesis of RA. RA synovial fibroblasts and "fibroblast-like synoviocytes" (FLS) play an important role in RA [6, 7].

Genetic and environmental factors are associated with RA. These factors include infectious agents, exposure to cigarette smoke, air pollution, insecticides, and occupational exposures to mineral oil and silica. But so far, smoking is the only environmental risk factor that has been extensively studied and widely accepted [3]. When environmental factors are considered some of them can be controlled, but the control of genetic and epigenetic regulation is highly complex and difficult to predict. The contribution of epigenetic gene regulation is considerably less well established. Epigenetics is a mechanism that regulates gene expression independently of the underlying DNA sequence. In early 2000s, with the discovery of micro RNAs (miRNAs), researchers have started to discuss their roles in physiological and pathologic processes [8]. miRNAs are small noncoding RNAs 18–25 nucleotides in length that block the translation or induce the degradation of target mRNA [9]. The clinical application of epigenomic information has improved in recent years. A growing body of evidence suggests that miRNAs participate in the inflammatory disorders including RA [10–12].

In this chapter, we summarize the biogenesis and function of miRNA, with an emphasis of its role in the pathogenesis and the importance of miRNA in RA as a potential biomarker.

2. What are microRNAs?

The small RNAs are crucial for the cellular gene regulatory systems. Over the last decade, these small RNAs have become important regulators in eukaryotic genomes. These noncoding RNAs regulate genes and genomes. This regulation includes chromatin structure, transcription, RNA processing, RNA stability, and translation. Generally, the small RNAs show inhibitory activity on gene expression. One type of these small RNAs is microRNAs [13].

MicroRNAs (miRNAs) are small endogenous noncoding RNAs [13]. In 1993, Ambros and his collaborators discovered the first miRNA, lin-4 from *Caenorhabditis elegans*. Researchers studied the postembryonic development of *C.elegans* and found two noncoding RNAs which were produced by lin-4 with complementary sequences to the 3′UTR (un-translated region) of lin-14 mRNA [14]. These small transcripts could bind the 3′UTR of lin-14 mRNA and decrease protein levels without affecting mRNA stability. In early 2000s, Reinhart (and) et al discovered the second miRNA, let-7, and following this discovery, more than a dozen miRNAs were found in plant and animal species in 2000s [15–18]. The name "microRNA" was first used in 2001, and papers published in science reported that there were up to 50 miRNAs [19–22]. The brief history of miRNAs is reviewed in **Figure 1**.

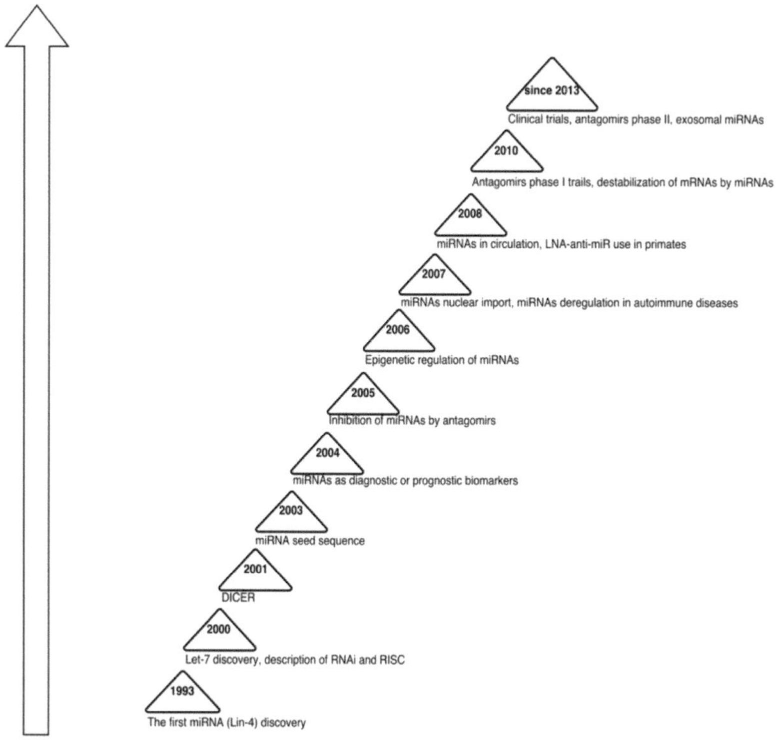

Figure 1. The brief history of miRNAs.

miRNAs are short (about 18–25 nucleotides long) noncoding RNAs that can affect messenger RNA (mRNA) processing at the post-transcriptional level [15]. They are endogenous and goal-oriented expressed products of an organism's own genome [13]. Chromosomal locations of miRNAs affect the expression and function themselves [23]. According to their genomic localizations, miRNAs can be classified into five groups [24]:

1. Intergenic miRNAs (miRNA genes are located between two consecutive protein-coding genes).
2. Intronic miRNAs in noncoding transcripts (miRNA genes are located in any intron of a noncoding RNA gene).
3. Intronic miRNAs in protein-coding transcripts (miRNA genes are located in any intron of a protein-coding RNA gene).
4. Exonic miRNAs in noncoding transcripts (miRNA genes are located in any exon of a noncoding RNA gene).
5. Exonic miRNAs in protein-coding transcripts (miRNA genes are located in any exon of a protein-coding RNA gene).

Some miRNAs are located in every second group because of alternative splicing [9]. Intergenic miRNAs are transcribed from their own promoters but intragenic miRNAs generally located in the same orientation as the host genes [24] (**Figure 2**).

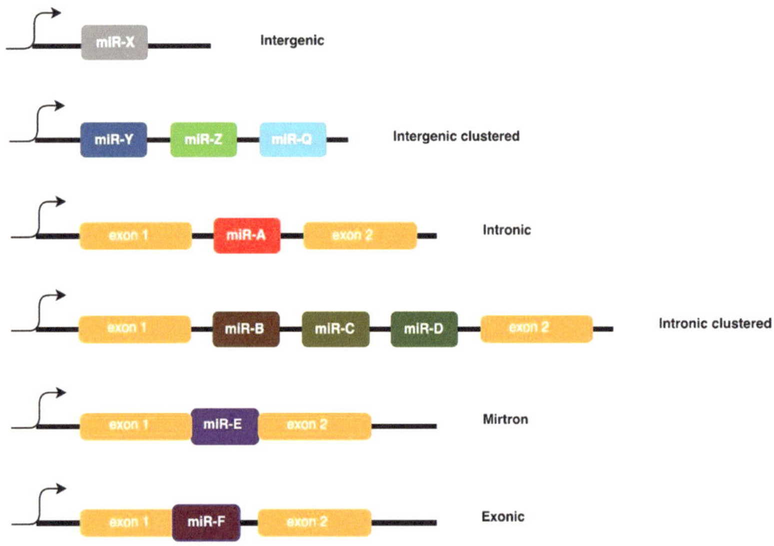

Figure 2. The genomic organization of miRNAs.

The scientific denomination rule is simple for the miRNAs. The mature miRNA is abbreviated with a capitalized "miR-" while the uncapitalized "mir-" indicates both the gene locus and precursor miRNA (pre-miRNA and pri-miRNA). Every miRNA is named according to discovery order, and "MIR" refers to the gene that encodes them. The numbering of miRNA genes is simply sequential. For example, miR-21 was discovered before the miR-155 [10]. In addition, three letters specific for each species precede each name. Thus "hsa-miR155" means that this miR origins from *Homo sapiens* while ggo-mir-155 is an example of gorilla's miRNA name. A letter after the number in the suffix is used to differentiate among multiple members of the same family (e.g., hsa-mir-155a and hsa-mir-155b). Today, miRNAs is still a popular subject for the researchers and have been studied in many organisms. Some miRNA databases (http://www.mirbase.org/, http://mirdb.org/miRDB/, http://www.microrna.org/microrna/home.do and so forth) are available and every moment the miRNA list is updated [25, 26].

3. miRNA biogenesis

In the early 2000s, the scientific world discovered small RNAs. They work as gene regulators, but their biogenesis is still unclear. Most mammalian miRNA genes are located in the intron region; some are located in the exon region and also approximately 30% are located in the intergenic regions. Since 2000, the miRNA biogenesis pathway has been studied and in 2001, Mello and his colleagues obtained the first data [17].

Generally, mammalian miRNA biogenesis pathway can be divided into two main parts with regard to processing pri-miRNAs: canonical and noncanonical [27]. In the canonical miRNA biogenesis pathway, the pri-miRNA is processed to pre-miRNA in the nucleus. In the noncanonical miRNA biogenesis pathway, mirtrons participate in microprocessor processing as alternative miRNA precursors. There are some differences between pri-miRNAs and mirtrons. Mirtrons arise from the spliced-out introns and lack lower stem loop structure and the flanking single-stranded segments thus the mirtrons bypass Drosha processing [28, 29].

The canonical miRNA biogenesis pathway is Drosha and Dicer dependent. Drosha is a member of ribonuclease III enzyme family, and the core nuclease that initiates miRNA processing in the nucleus [16]. Dicer is also a member of RNAse III family. It cleaves double-stranded RNA (ds-RNA) and precursor miRNA (pre-miRNA) into short dsRNA fragments. Dicer forms the mature miRNA in the cytoplasm [16, 18]. The noncanonical miRNA biogenesis pathway is Drosha independent/Dicer dependent. Here, microprocessor is not required. Mirtrons are a type of miRNA that are direct Dicer substrates. A number of noncanonical pathways have been described, but most pathways remain unclear. Besides, mirtrons comprise small part of the miRNAs, so generally miRNAs are processed via canonical pathway [16, 18, 27].

Microprocessor components, Drosha, DiGeorge critical region 8 (DGCR8, also known as Pasha), and Dicer, are essential for the canonical miRNA biogenesis, and the biogenesis pathway is compartmentalized and stepwise [27]. The canonical mRNA biogenesis pathway starts with RNA Pol II-mediated transcription of genomic region containing miRNA genes. Transcripts (pri-miRNAs) are capped (at the 5′ end) and polyadenylated (at the 3′ end). The pri-miRNAs are cleaved to pre-miRNA hairpins by RNAse III enzyme Drosha in the nucleus. DGCR8 (Pasha) proteins accompany this processing. Then, pre-miRNAs are exported from the nucleus to cytoplasm by exportin-5 (XPO-5) via Ran-GTP–dependent mechanism. In the cytoplasm, pre-miRNA is processed into a mature miRNA. RNAse III Dicer cleaves the pre-miRNA together with trans-activation response RNA binding protein (TRBP)/protein activator of PKR (PACT) proteins to produce unstable, 18–22 nt asymmetric miRNA:miRNA* duplex.

miRNA represents guide RNA strand, and the other miRNA* means passenger RNA strand. The guide RNA strand incorporates into RNA-induced silencing complex (RISC), and passenger RNA strand is discarded. Argonaute (AGO) is one of the key components of RISC for this process [18, 27]. The canonical miRNA biogenesis pathway is summarized in **Figure 3**.

The alternative miRNA biogenesis pathways are named noncanonical pathways. These pathways do not require all enzymes and protein factors of the canonical pathway. Some miRNAs differ from the others in terms of structure and function and these miRNAs bypass one or more steps of miRNA canonical biogenesis [27, 29]. Dicer is required for both pathways—canonical and noncanonical, but Drosha and DGCR8 are only needed for the canonical pathway. If there is a mutation or deficiency of these enzymes, miRNA biogenesis goes on via the noncanonical pathway. The noncanonical miRNA biogenesis pathway can be divided mainly into two classes [27, 30].

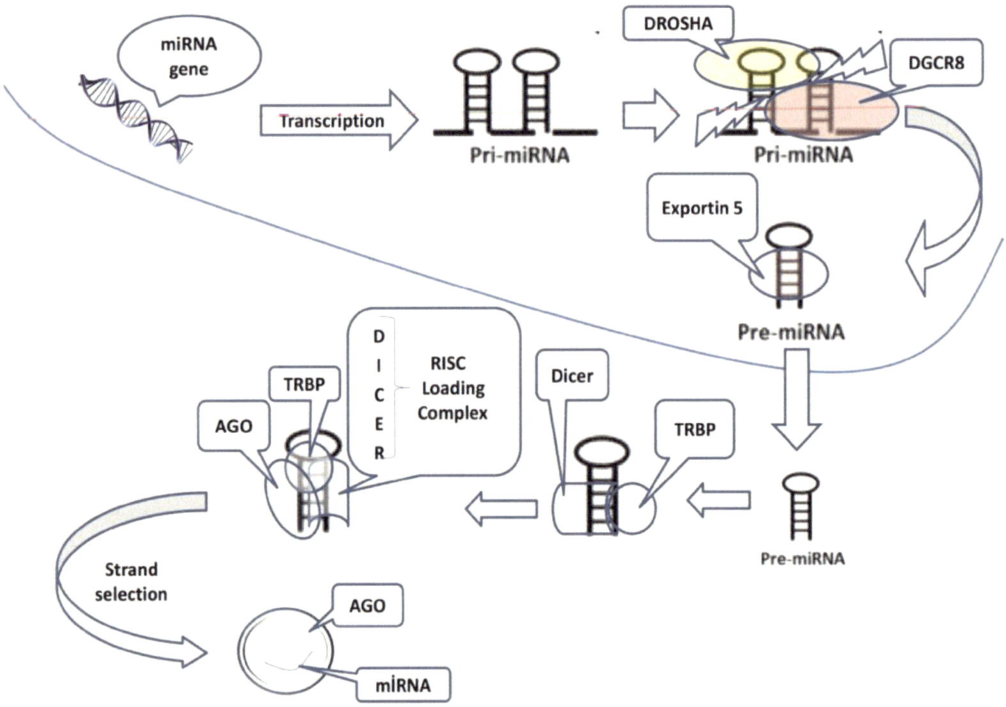

Figure 3. The canonical miRNA biogenesis pathway.

3.1. Drosha/DGCR8-independent/Dicer-dependent pathways

3.1.1. Mirtron pathway

Some introns form short RNA hairpins, and they are termed "mirtrons" that can be spliced resulting in a nonlinear intermediate. Investigations of the data of small RNAs from Drosophila melanogaster and Caenohabditis elegans led to the discovery of mirtrons [28]. They can be debranched into pre-miRNA hairpins and form the duplex. After this step, this product can join he (the) canonical pathway and is ready to be transported to the cytoplasm by exportin-5 (EXP-5) [29].

Depending on the splice donor and acceptor site, mirtrons can be categorized into three groups: 5′-tailed mirtron, regular mirtron, and 3′-tailed mirtron. Generally, 3′-tailed mirtrons have been found in Drosophila, and 5′-tailed mirtrons have only been described in vertebrates [28, 29]. Mirtrons being a new research area, there are many unanswered questions.

3.1.2. snoRNA-derived RNAs (sdRNAs)

Small-nucleolar RNAs are a class of noncoding RNAs. Generally, they show similar properties and structures to miRNAs. They are dependent on Dicer and can be bound with AGO acting as a miRNA [29, 31].

3.1.3. *miRNAs from tdRNAs*

The first (tdRNA) tRNA-derived RNA species to be discovered were isoleucine tRNA-derived miRNA [27]. Normally, they differ from regular miRNAs but they have RNA silencing function. tRNA-derived (tdRNA) precursors can be a potential substrate of Dicer because of their different folding form [29, 31]. In the light of this information, they have different properties from typical mammalian miRNAs, and their pattern of behavior remains a puzzle.

3.1.4. *miRNAs from endogenous short hairpin RNAs (shRNAs)*

Several studies have shown that some shRNAs could join the noncanonical miRNA-processing pathway. Normally, in the canonical miRNA pathway, pre-miRNAs hairpins are conserved and thus can be recognized by microprocessor complex. However, shRNA-derived miRNAs do not have the microprocessor sequence. For this reason, they are DiGeorge critical region-8 (DGCR-8) independent [27, 29]

3.2. Drosha/DGCR8-dependent/Dicer-independent pathways

Some miRNAs mature in a different way. One of them is miR-451. MiR-451 maturation occurs without Dicer. Initially, pri-miR-451 is cleaved by Drosha/DGCR8 to form pre-miRNA duplex. But it is too short to present to Dicer as a substrate, so directly it interacts with AGO proteins [29, 31]. The miRNA biogenesis pathways and their regulation have been studied extensively in last 10 years, but further information is required for miRNA processing.

4. miRNA function

The functions of miRNAs are post-transcriptional repression and degradation of mRNAs [13]. They have different expression patterns and regulate several biological and pathological processes [16, 32, 33]. The major function of miRNAs is protein synthesis inhibition. They can maintain this function either by inhibition of translation or by mRNA degradation [34, 35]. The miRNA-mRNA interaction is important for miRNA function, and each mature miRNA interacts with specific miRNA/miRNAs. Generally, the interaction takes place between the miRNA seed region and 3′ UTR of mRNA for the inhibition of target mRNA. There are a few exceptions about miRNA binding sites. In some cases, the miRNA-mRNA interaction occurs at the 5′-UTR. The second issue is miRNA's tissue specificity. MiRNAs are expressed in a tissue-specific fashion, and also, the action of miRNA is tissue specific [36–39].

Identification of miRNA target genes is crucial for the functional characterization of miRNAs. Recently, we can predict the target gene with the help of some bioinformatics algorithms and software. The most popular software is TargetScan [5, 10]. If *in silico* analysis is insufficient, further analysis can be needed. Some genetic or biochemical methods are preferable. The success of the prediction is important to understand miRNA function.

The miRNAs have a part as an adaptor for miRISC to recognize and regulate target mRNAs. MiRISC regulates the translation of AGO proteins by introducing silencing through mRNA deadenylation, degradation, or translation [13]. miRNAs which are integrated into the RISC complex control the gene expression the level of post-transcription by reducing miRNA stability or inhibiting translation of mRNA [9, 32, 40]. Besides, miRNAs can affect several epigenetic regulators (DNA methyltransferases and histone deacetylases) [16].

In addition to mRNAs repression, some miRNAs have positive effects on gene expression [9]. This can occur directly or indirectly. For instance, miR-373 binds to the promoter of E-cadherin directly and increases the function of RNA polymerase. If its target mRNA does not consist of poly (A)-tail, AGO2 activates the gene expression [8, 9].

The selectivity in gene regulation mechanism depends on the degree of the match occurred between target mRNA and miRNA. Exact match is usually found in plants. miRISC complex which make partial matches is required to make an exact match with the seed region in the related to miRNA to inhibit the translation [41, 42]. Although many miRNAs cause of gene silencing by reducing the target mRNA stability, some miRNAs lead to gene silencing by inhibiting target mRNA translation, but there is not enough evidence about what stage they repress. In general, studies suggest that miRNAs repress the translation with four different mechanisms: (1) suppression of protein synthesis, (2) a drop of premature mRNAs in ribosomes, (3) slowing down during the alongation step of protein synthesis, (4) in parallel with protein synthesis the fragmentation of protein [40, 43, 44].

The function of miRNAs has been studied since the first two microRNAs discovered. miRNAs are considered key regulators to physiological processes, such as cellular and tissue differentiation, apoptosis, innate, and adaptive immune responses and development [13, 17, 35, 45, 46]. Thus, miRNAs are crucial for the regulation of biological processes [17]. Deregulation of this regulatory network can lead to the initiation of undesired pathological processes, such as cancer, fibrotic diseases, and autoimmune diseases [17, 35, 45, 46].

miRNAs have essential roles in immune system as they arrange innate and adaptive immune systems and have pivotal roles in the regulation of inflammation, by controlling the differentiation of B cells, conventional T cells, and regulatory T cells [11, 39].

4.1. Innate immunity and miRNAs

The innate immune system fights microorganisms. It has many cell types, which are physical epithelial barriers, phagocytic leukocytes, dendritic cells, natural killer (NK) cells, and circulating plasma proteins. Pattern recognition receptors (PRRs) recognize microorganisms and include toll-like receptors (TLRs), C-type lectin-like receptors (CLRs), retinoic acid-inducible gene (RIG)-I-like-receptors (RLRs) and nucleotide-binding oligomerization domain (NOD)-like receptors (NLRs). This process starts to intracellular signaling pathways. TLR has 10 subtypes such as TLR1, TLR2, TRL3, TLR4, TLR5, TLR6, TRL7, TRL8, TRL9, and TLR10 [47–50]. TLR4 identify lipopolysaccharides (LPSs). miR-146a/b, miR-132, and miR-155 are overexpressed for the LPS-mediated inflammatory responses. miR-146 upregulation causes interleukin-1 receptor-associated kinase (IRAK) 1 and genes expression and tumor necrosis factors receptor–associated factor (TRAF) 6 [51]. miR-146 was investigated in *in vitro* model of mouse macrophages, and it is a negative regulator of IRAK1, IRAK2 and TRAF6 [52]. On the other hand, miR-155 and miR-125b levels are related to TNF-α secretion in mouse macrophages. Regulation of miR-155 and miR-125b is LPS/TNF-α dependent; therefore, it is suggested that they are new targets of drug design. miR-155 increases TNF-α translation, Fas-associated death domain protein (FADD), IkappaB kinase epsilon (IKKepsilon), and TNFR superfamily-interacting serine–threonine kinase 1 (Ripk1) [53]. One study showed that miR-147 increased in murine macrophages after stimulation with TLR2, TLR3, and TLR4 ligands and in the lungs of mice after LPS exposure [54]. Also, NF-κB is regulated by miR-1303. Mir-1303 regulates the process of autophagy related to mycobacteria by targeting Atg2B [55]. Besides, miR-146a and miR-155 affect IFN-type I synthesis by TLR-7 and TLR-9, some miRNAs such as miR-126, miR-21, miR-146a, miR-155, and miR-1246 can mediate regulation with epigenetic modification [56].

4.2. Adaptive immunity and miRNAs

T and B-lymphocytes are major cellular components of the adaptive immunity. As previously described, Dicer enzymes are important in the biogenesis of miRNA. In B cells, miR-181b and miR-148a play role as miR-148a inhibits the expression of the autoimmune suppressor Gadd45α [57, 58]. In T cell early development, decrease of Dicer leads to reduction of T cell numbers both in the thymus and peripheral lymphoid organs [59]. In early B cell development, miR-17 deficiency induced by ablation of Dicer in pro-B cells affected B cell antibody diversity and B cell survival [60]. miR-326 and miR-155 are related to IL-17 [61]. Moreover, miR-155 expression related to Th17 cell production and miR-155 downregulated the LPS-induced inflammatory process [62, 63]. miR-146 has an essential role in the adaptive immune system. In the Treg cells miR-146 is an activator of STAT1 transcription that is associated with Th1-mediated autoimmunity [64].

Many studies in animal (many researches on animal olabilir) models and clinical studies showed that miRNAs participate in the inflammation and autoimmune diseases mechanisms. In humans, loss of miRNA expression related of the many autoimmune conditions. Especially, multiple sclerosis (MS), osteoarthritis, and rheumatoid arthritis (RA) are most studied (are the most).

5. Expression profiles of miRNAs in rheumatoid arthritis patients

RA, characterized by chronic joint inflammation, is an autoimmune disease. Small joints of the hands and feet are affected most (more or the most) often; however, the disease is known to vary among individuals. In the general population, RA affects roughly three times more women (females) than men (males) and is more common between 35 and 50 years and in older individuals [65–68]. Persistent inflammation over time leads to joint damage and disability [69]. This disease is characterized by autoimmunity with multiple joint lesions and systemic inflammation. Also, patients can develop complications, which result in lifelong disability and increased mortality. Accordingly, RA is a growing public health concern as it is associated with significant social and economic burden [70].

In genetically susceptible people, various environmental factors can act as a trigger for inducing autoimmunity [71]. Recent experimental data showed that the pathogenesis of RA is associated with epigenetic regulation. Over the past few years, it has become clear that different microRNAs (miRNAs) expression levels, particularly in RA, contribute to the development of autoimmunity. miRNAs plays (play) multiple roles in regulation of pro-inflammatory cytokine secretion and development of immune cells, and they work in the induction or suppression of autoimmunity and ECM remodeling. Thus, dysregulated miRNA expression seems to promote the molecular mechanisms of the RA process [72–77]. Stanczyk et al. described for the first time the dysregulation of miRNAs in RA in 2008 [78]. They reported increased miR-155 and miR-146a expression in RA synovial fibroblasts compared to those in osteoarthritis (OA) patients. miRNAs expression is detected in several cell types in RA, and miRNAs expression profiles can regulate many physiological actions in RA (**Table 1**) [79, 80].

Cell type	**miRNA**		**Refs.**
	Downregulated	**Upregulated**	
Synovial tissue	miR-22	miR-146a	[80–86]
	miR-23b	miR-146b	
	miR-30a	miR-150	
		miR-155	
		miR-223	
Synovial fibroblasts	miR-124a	miR-133a	[85–91]
	miR-34a	miR-142-3p	
	miR-22	miR-142-5p	
	miR-152	miR-146a	
	miR-375	miR-155	
		miR-203	
		miR-221	
		miR-222	
		miR-323-3p	
Synovial fluid	miR-152	miR-16	[86, 92, 93]
	miR-375	miR-146a	
		miR-155	
		miR-223	
Synovium macrophages		miR-146a miR-155	[81, 94]
Whole blood		miR-99	[95, 96]
		miR-100	
		miR-125b	
		miR-146a	

Cell type	miRNA		Refs.
	Downregulated	Upregulated	
		miR-155	
Peripheral blood mononuclear cells (PBMCs)	miR-21	miR-26a	[82, 96–98]
		miR-132	
		miR-146a	
		miR-146b	
		miR-150	
		miR-155	
		miR-16	
Plasma and serum	miR-16	miR-16	[91, 95, 98–100]
	miR-125a-3p	miR-21	
	miR-126-3p	miR-24	
	miR-132	miR-26a	
	miR-146a	miR-125a-5p	
	miR-155	miR-125b	
		miR-126-3p	
		miR-223	
		miR-451	

Table 1. Expression of miRNAs in RA.

6. The roles of miRNAs in RA

Several miRNAs are found to be upregulated or downregulated in synovial tissue and cells of joint or blood compartment of patients with RA. The bone and joint destruction occurring in RA is accompanied by specific changes in cellular miRNAs that can affect epigenetic regulation. The current literature demonstrates that a variety of miRNAs is frequently dysregulated in RA patients.

miR-15/miR-16: miR-15a/16-1 and miR-15b/16-2 are highly protected in mammalian species. miR-15a is downregulated in arthritic synovial tissue, which has a potential role in apoptosis [95]. Nagata et al showed that in synovium miR15a, expression levels are lower in diseased mice than in healthy controls [101]. miR-15 plays a role in apoptosis; it has a negative regulatory effect on Bcl-2. Sera of patients with early RA show differential levels of miR-16-1 and miR-16-2, which are increased in peripheral blood mononuclear cells (PBMC) of RA patients [86, 95, 98]. Besides, miR-16 is a good candidate as a marker of disease activity. It is one of the key pro-inflammatory (proinflammatory) mediators in RA: mir-16 being able to target "tumor necrosis factor-α" (TNF-α) may be the biomarker of the RA.

miR-17-92 cluster: It is a controller of apoptosis, lots of research groups found de-regulated expression of miRNAs within this cluster in the context of RA [102].

miR-18: miR18a is upregulated in fibroblast-like synoviocytes (FLS) of RA patients. It is important in inflammation, because miR-18 contributes to NFκBmediated cartilage destruction and chronic inflammation in the joint through a positive feedback loop involving silencing of the "nuclear factor kappa-light-chain-enhancer of activated B cells" (NFκB) inhibitor TNFinduced protein-3 [103].

miR-21: In RA patients, levels of miR-21 are raised in plasma [99]; on the other hand, one study showed that miR-21 level is decreased in peripheral blood mononuclear cells (PBMCs). Downregulation of miR-21 is related to upregulation of "signal transducer and activator of transcription 3" (STAT-3) expression and decreased "forkhead box P3" (FOXP 3) mRNA levels in RA patients [104].

miR-22: Lin and his colleagues showed that expression of miR-22 is down regulated and negatively correlated with Cyr61 expression in synovial tissue of RA patients [85]. CYR61 expression is high in RA FLS and stimulates RA synovial fibroblast proliferation and interleukin (IL)-6 secretion in an autocrine-paracrine manner [85]. CYR61 may encourage synovial tissue hyperplasia alongside IL-6-dependent Th17 differentiation, which is critical for joint lesions in RA.

miR-23b: miR-23b is reported to be decreased in RA. miR-23b expression level is reduced and correlated with the high concentration of IL-17 in tissue samples from RA patients [83]. IL-17 suppresses the expression of miR-23b in human primary FLS. miR-23b regulates IL-1β, TNF-α, and IL-17 signaling and decreased levels of miR-23b in RA may be responsible for the induction of autoimmune inflammation.

miR-24: In RA, increased levels of plasma miR-24 have been reported, also its level significantly increased compared to OA [100]. Furin enzyme is important for the processing of latent TGF-β1, which may increase the inflammation by miR-24. Furin is a protein that is encoded by the FUR gene in humans. It was named FUR because it is in the upstream region of FES oncogene. Furin is also known as paired basic amino acid cleaving enzyme (PACE).

miR-26a: Murata and Nimoto worked with this molecule, and they showed that miR-26a is overexpressed in PBMCs and plasma of RA patients. Thus, it may be biomarker for the diagnosis of RA [82, 100]. miR-26a is upregulated during differentiation of IL-17 and generation of CD4+ cells. CD4+ cells are very important in the pathology of RA [82].

miR27a and miR27b: These miRNAs' expression is decreased in OA chondrocytes and coincides with increased expression of "Insulin Like Growth Factor Binding Protein 5" (IGFBP5) and Matrix Metallopeptidase-13 (MMP13) [105, 106].

miR-30a: miR-30a has been shown to be downregulated in RA synovial tissue and miR-30a-3p has a critical role in the regulation of "B lymphocyte activating factor of the tumor necrosis factor family" (BAFF) expression, which has a major impact in the regulation of the autoimmune responses occurring in RA [107].

miR-34a/miR-34b: miR-34a and miR-34b family are investigated in RA. miR34a is downregulated in RA synovial fibroblasts. The "X-linked inhibitor of apoptosis protein" (XIAP) is identified as a direct target of miR-34a [89]. So, miR-24 may contribute to the impaired apoptosis of activated RA synovial fibroblasts. On the other hand, miR-34b is overexpressed in RA T cells.

miR-124a: In 2009, Nakamachi et al. identified decreased expression levels of miR-124 in RA FLS. They showed that miR-24a targets the "monocyte chemoattractant protein-1" (MCP-1) mRNA expression and "cyclin-dependent kinase-2" (CDK-2) and decreases their protein levels [88]. miR-124 controls inflammatory process in RA, indirectly. The curtailed expression of miR-124a can contribute to RA pathogenesis via increased RA synovial fibroblast proliferation, angiogenesis, and leukocyte chemotaxis [89].

miR-125a-3p/miR-125a-5p/miR-125b: The family of miR-125 is dysregulated in the peripheral blood of RA patients. Kim et al. found that miR-125a-5p and miR-125b activate the pro-inflammatory NF-κB signaling pathway [108]. Thus, they may have roles in the induction of excessive inflammation in RA. Because of that, miRNA levels are monitored in serum from RA patients [95]. MiR-125b has a specific role in the regulation of normal and abnormal immune functions. Hruskova et al. suggested that the expression of miR-125b in those patients may present a novel biomarker for monitoring the treatment outcome during the early phase of RA [109].

miR-126-3p: miR-126-3p is significantly irregular in the plasma of RA patients. There is conflicting evidence regarding miR-126-3p. Wang et al. showed that miR-126-3p is lower in the plasma of RA patients [99], while another research group showed that the expression level of circulated miR-126-3p is markedly elevated in RA [100]. miR-126 can inhibit PI3K/AKT signaling pathway. It may clinically be helpful for RA patients [110].

miR-132: The expression of miR-132 of PBMCs from RA patients was twice higher as compared to controls [45]. However, miR-132 concentrations were found to be lower in RA plasma than in the plasma of healthy individuals [86]. Plasma concentrations of miR-132 differentiated patients with RA or OA from healthy controls, though plasma and synovial fluid miR-132 failed to differentiate RA from OA. Besides, plasma miR-132 or its SF/PB ratio (ratio of concentration of synovial fluid miRNA to plasma miRNA) correlated with tender joint count. These results indicate that miR-132 may have a role in systemic conditions with joint inflammation, such as RA [86]. miR-132 studies have mainly focused on central nervous system and neurotransmission; however, further analyses are required to determine the importance of miR-132 in inflammatory diseases [111].

miR-133a: MiR-133a is upregulated in RA synovial fibroblasts. Also, miR-133a is known as a negative regulator of the "Runt-related transcription factor 2" (Runx2), which is essential for the osteoblast differentiation [112].

miR146a/miR-146b: Studies showed that miR-146 is upregulated in all RA samples. One study found an increased basal expression of miR-146a in RA synovial fibroblasts compared with OA synovial fibroblasts [81, 87, 113]. In addition, increased expression levels of miR-146a have been observed in synovial fluid [85, 86, 97], synovial tissue [82, 83, 99], PBMCs [96, 97, 99, 114, 115], and whole blood [96] of RA patients. Expression of miR-146a is detected in many cell types, T cells, B cells, monocytes, macrophages, and IL-17 producing CD4+ cells [81, 82, 97, 114, 115]. However, plasma or serum miR-146a levels in patients with RA are comparable to that seen in healthy controls [86, 98], and two studies demonstrated that miR-146a was markedly decreased in plasma from patients with established RA [99]. miR-146a can inhibit T-helper 1-mediated responses and is required for the suppressive activity of Treg cells, which are both important in RA pathogenesis [64, 115]. Nevertheless, the increasing expression of miR-146a is not specific to RA, as it is also reported in OA cartilage after stimulation by IL-1b [116].

Pauley and Abou-Zeid found that peripheral blood mononuclear cell expression of miR-146a was positively correlated with CRP, ESR, DAS28 index, and TNF-α concentration [97, 115]. There are two known gene targets of miR-146a, that is, TNF-α/TNF receptor-associated factor 6 (TRAF6) and IL-1 receptor-associated kinase 1 (IRAK1). Also, miRNA-146a can regulate genes such as FAF1, IRAK2, FADD, IRF-5, STAT-1, and PTC-1. However, miR-146a has also been reported to correlate inversely with the tender joint count [97, 115]. In addition, miRNA-146a expression levels in the peripheral blood of RA patients were comparable to the levels seen in synovial tissue and fibroblastic cells of those patients [97]. miR-146a/b is induced in response to a variety of microbial components and pro-inflammatory cytokines, such as LPS, CpG, IFN-β, and TNF-α [51]. miR-146a in PBMCs enhances the function of Th1 cells and induces the expression of TNF-α, MCP-1, and NFκB p65 [117]. miR-146b was reported to increase in RA synovial tissue and in PBMCs of RA patients [82]. Upregulated miR-146b is related with infiltration of IL-17-producing T cells in RA synovium and higher expression of IL-17 within T cells expanded from RA PBMCs. So, it suggested that miR-146a and miR-146b are strongly implicated in RA development.

miR-152: Decreased expression of miR152 is reported in FLS of arthritic rats. It leads to activation of the Wnt-signaling pathway through direct targeting of "DNA (cytosine-5)-methyltransferase-1" DNMT1 and "encoding Frizzled8" (FZD8) by turn [92, 93].

miR-155: This is the most widely studied miRNA in RA. miR-155 expression profiles in RA synovial fibroblasts can also be induced by TNF-α [118]. The first miRNAs found to be abnormally expressed in FLS with RA were miR146a and miR155, both previously known as important regulators of inflammation. Also, miR146a and miR155 are two miRNAs, which are negative and positive regulators of inflammatory responses, respectively. miR-155 has been shown to express strongly in RA synovial tissue, synovial fluid and synovial fluid CD14+ cells [118]. Nonetheless, miR-155 concentrations are significantly lower as compared to controls in RA serum [98, 99]. The increased level of miR-155 in synovial fluid CD14+ cells and in synovial tissue macrophages is associated with decreased expression of the miR-155 target, a potent inhibitor of inflammation, called Src homology 2-containing inositol phosphatase-1 (SHIP-1), in patients with RA [94]. In addition, targets of miR-155 are the genes ZNF652, matrix metalloproteinase (MMP)-1 MMP-3, SHIP-1, c-Maf, PU.1, CEBP, ZIC3, HIVEP2, ARID2, SMAD5, and Bach-1. These pathways are all play a role in RA.

miR-203: One study showed that miR-203 is higher in RA synovial fluid in comparison with OA synovial fluid. Expression of miR-203 in the RA and OA synovium may be explained by differences in cellular composition of synovial tissue among RA patients [67, 78, 91]. Overexpression of miR-203 in RA synovial fluid resulted in higher release of MMP-1 and secretion of IL-6 via the NF-κB pathway and NF-κB-dependent production of IL-6, thus contributing to the RA synovial fluid activated phenotype and joint inflammatory state. Also, miR-203 plays a role in oncogenic transformation, proliferation, migration, and invasiveness of tumor cells. This mechanism is unknown in RA.

miR-221/miR-222: miR-221 and miR-222 are expressed together. miR-221/miR-222 are overexpressed in synovial fluids, blood serum, and synovial tissues of RA patients. MiR-221 plays a role in increasing production of pro-inflammatory cytokines, RA synovial fibroblast activation and migration. It also has a role in increasing resistance to apoptosis [119].

miR-223: miR223 is increased in T cells from patients with RA compared to levels in T cells from healthy donors [120]. miR-223 overexpressed in peripheral blood CD3+ and CD4+ naive T-lymphocytes of RA patients contributes to pathogenesis of the disease. CD14+ monocytes from RA synovia also overexpress miR223 and modulate differentiation of myeloid precursors into osteoclasts [121].

miR-323-3p: miR-323-3p expression is higher in RA synovial fibroblasts than OA synovial fibroblasts [90]. This miRNA may increase the Wnt-cadherin pathway and decrease the levels of target protein "β-transducin repeat containing E3 ubiquitin protein ligase" (BTRC) that contains an inhibitor of β-catenin [90]. It has been shown that miR-323-3p may have proinflammatory role in RA.

miR-375: miR-375 regulates the pathogenesis of adjuvant-induced arthritis rat model through the canonical Wnt signaling pathway [93].

miR-451: miR451, most preserved in vertebrates, regulates cell proliferation, invasion, and apoptosis. Neutrophils are important players in RA pathogenesis. miR451, significantly overexpressed in RA serum, peripheral blood T cells from patients with active RA and downregulated in neutrophils from patients with RA. Besides, it negatively regulates the migration of neutrophils by silencing CPNE3 (encoding copine3) and RAB5A (encoding Rasrelated protein Rab5A) [122]. In RA, miR-451 may reduce neutrophil chemotaxis through p38 MAPK (p38 mitogen-activated protein kinases) [122].

miR-455-3p: miR-455-3p can drive cartilage degradation by suppressing the expression of key molecules involved in cartilage formation. Increased expression of miR4553p in OA cartilage contributes to its destruction by targeting ACVR2B (encoding activin receptor type2B), SMAD2 (encoding MAD homology 2), CHRDL1 (encoding chordinlike protein 1), and by suppressing TGF-β signaling [118].

miR-498: miR-498 is associated with neurotransmission and inflammation. miR-498 is downregulated in CD4+ T cells from synovial fluid and peripheral blood [85].

miR-886-3p: A recent study reported that the combination of low expression of miR-22 and high expression of miR-886-3p were predictive of a good clinical response to adalimumab treatment in patients with early RA [123].

7. The importance of miRNAs in RA

MicroRNAs (miRNAs) are involved in the pathophysiological mechanisms underlying human diseases states. During the last decade, researchers have obtained a growing body of evidence regarding miRNAs in many human autoimmune diseases, such as RA, multiple sclerosis, psoriasis and systemic lupus erythematosus. miRNAs-mediated regulation is very clear from all of the present data and can play an important role in the development of various inflammatory conditions. So, dysregulation of miRNA expression (loss or downregulation of miRNA because of mutation, miRNA promoter region mutation, or overexpression of miRNA, epigenetic activation etc.) can lead to a variety of diseases.

For example, upregulation of miR-146 and miR-203 were observed in psoriasis [11]. Also, serum miR-1266 levels were highly significant in patients with psoriasis [124, 125]. Aberrations of miR-223, miR-143, miR-142, miR-378, miR-100, miR-21, and miR-31 levels were also found in these patients [126–128]. In systemic lupus erythematosus, some miRNAs, miR-146, miR-17-5p, miR-112, miR-141, miR-184, miR-196a, miR-383, and miR-409-3p, are downregulated, but miR-21, miR-61, miR-78, miR-142-3, miR-189, miR-198, miR-298, miR-299-3p, and miR-342 are upregulated in PBMCS from patients as compared to healthy controls [11, 127–131]. In multiple sclerosis, miR-18b, miR-599, and miR-96 are dysregulated in PBMCs in those patients [11, 132].

RA is a polygenic disease with multiple effects and miRNAs are post-transcriptional regulators of gene expression. In RA, high miRNA expressions (high mirna expressions mı olacak?) have been identified in different sites and cells, such as synovial tissue, synovial fibroblasts, PBMCs, plasma, synovial fluid, and activated immune cells within injured joints. The identified miRNA candidates for RA play a substantial role for key molecular mechanisms. These mechanisms are especially cytokine signaling pathways and inflammation. So, miRNAs are upregulated or downregulated in RA patients, relative to other diseases and healthy controls.

miRNAs, as diagnostic tools for RA, have many advantages. As such, miRNAs are stable and can be isolated from different parts of bodies (synovial fibroblasts, blood, plasma). miRNAs can be detected in circulating blood without the need for biopsies. Finally, miRNAs expression levels can be estimated by PCR.

8. Conclusion and perspectives

Since the discovery that microRNAs (miRNAs) take part in biological and pathological processes, it has become important to determine the roles.

In this chapter, we have summarized the role of miRNAs in RA. RA is a systemic autoimmune disorder characterized by chronic inflammation of the synovial tissue, and many studies suggest that miRNAs play role on autoimmunity in RA, as miR-16, miR-146b, miR-132, and miR-155 are upregulated in RA circulation. This suggests that miRNAs contribute to

RA pathogenesis. miR-124a is downregulated in RA synovium tissue [88] while miR-146a, miR-155 and miR-203 are upregulated in RA synovium tissue [51, 91, 133]. As we mentioned above, miR-146 and miR-203 are also upregulated in psoriasis; for this reason, they are questionable as possible biomarkers. miR-16, miR-132, miR-146, and miR-155 are upregulated in RA PBMCs, and miR-223 is upregulated in CD4+ naïve T-lymphocytes of RA patients [121].

Recently, the understanding of the molecular mechanism, prediction, or identification of miRNA targets is the main subjects of research in this area. This contribution may be lead to consider miRNAs as therapeutic targets. However, some miRNAs mentioned above are not specific for RA, as they are also dysregulated in the other immune disorders or cancers.

In the past few years, some experimental models have been used to study the therapeutic potential of miRNAs in RA, but still they are insufficient. Further studies are necessary.

In summary, each miRNA that is identified for RA opens the door slightly in terms of diagnostic and/or prognostic marker. Today, the available evidence shows that miRNAs are not diagnostic markers yet, but they can be used for therapy in the future.

Author details

Merih Birlik[1*], Ayşe Koçak[2] and Duygu Harmancı[2]

*Address all correspondence to: birlikm@gmail.com

1 Department of Internal Medicine, Division of Rheumatology, Faculty of Medicine, Dokuz Eylül University, Izmir, Turkey

2 Department of Molecular Medicine, Graduate School of Health Sciences, Dokuz Eylül University, Izmir, Turkey

References

[1] Klareskog, L., A.I. Catrina, and S. Paget, *Rheumatoid arthritis.* Lancet, 2009. **373**(9664): p. 659–72.

[2] Scott, D.L., F. Wolfe, and T.W. Huizinga, *Rheumatoid arthritis.* Lancet, 2010. **376**(9746): p. 1094–108.

[3] Chung, I.M., et al., *Rheumatoid arthritis: The stride from research to clinical practice.* Int J Mol Sci, 2016. **17**(6).

[4] Akar, S., et al., *The prevalence of rheumatoid arthritis in an urban population of Izmir-Turkey.* Clin Exp Rheumatol, 2004. **22**(4): p. 416–20.

[5] McInnes, I.B. and G. Schett, *The pathogenesis of rheumatoid arthritis.* N Engl J Med, 2011. **365**(23): p. 2205–19.

[6] Vicente, R., et al., *Deregulation and therapeutic potential of microRNAs in arthritic diseases.* Nat Rev Rheumatol, 2016. **12**(4): p. 211–20.

[7] Turner, J.D. and A. Filer, *The role of the synovial fibroblast in rheumatoid arthritis pathogenesis.* Curr Opin Rheumatol, 2015. **27**(2): p. 175–82.

[8] Lai, E.C., *microRNAs: runts of the genome assert themselves.* Curr Biol, 2003. **13**(23): p. R925–36.

[9] Carthew, R.W. and E.J. Sontheimer, *Origins and mechanisms of miRNAs and siRNAs.* Cell, 2009. **136**(4): p. 642–55.

[10] Ceribelli, A., et al., *MicroRNAs in rheumatoid arthritis.* FEBS Lett, 2011. **585**(23): p. 3667–74.

[11] Furer, V., et al., *The role of microRNA in rheumatoid arthritis and other autoimmune diseases.* Clin Immunol, 2010. **136**(1): p. 1–15.

[12] Duroux-Richard, I., et al., *MicroRNAs as new player in rheumatoid arthritis.* Joint Bone Spine, 2011. **78**(1): p. 17–22.

[13] He, L. and G.J. Hannon, *MicroRNAs: Small RNAs with a big role in gene regulation.* Nat Rev Genet, 2004. **5**(7): p. 522–31.

[14] Lee, R.C., R.L. Feinbaum, and V. Ambros, *The C. elegans heterochronic gene lin-4 encodes small RNAs with antisense complementarity to lin-14.* Cell, 1993. **75**(5): p. 843–54.

[15] Almeida, M.I., R.M. Reis, and G.A. Calin, *MicroRNA history: discovery, recent applications, and next frontiers.* Mutat Res, 2011. **717**(1–2): p. 1–8.

[16] Bhaskaran, M. and M. Mohan, *MicroRNAs: history, biogenesis, and their evolving role in animal development and disease.* Vet Pathol, 2014. **51**(4): p. 759–74.

[17] Orellana, E.A. and A.L. Kasinski, *MicroRNAs in cancer: a historical perspective on the path from discovery to therapy.* Cancers (Basel), 2015. **7**(3): p. 1388–405.

[18] Riaz, A., R. Dalziel, V.M. Venturina, M.A. Shah, *MicroRNAs: History, biogenesis and modes of action to regulate gene expression.* Veterinaria, 2015. **2**: p. 14–20.

[19] Ruvkun, G., *Molecular biology. Glimpses of a tiny RNA world.* Science, 2001. **294**(5543): p. 797–9.

[20] Lagos-Quintana, M., et al., *Identification of novel genes coding for small expressed RNAs.* Science, 2001. **294**(5543): p. 853–8.

[21] Lau, N.C., et al., *An abundant class of tiny RNAs with probable regulatory roles in Caenorhabditis elegans.* Science, 2001. **294**(5543): p. 858–62.

[22] Lee, R.C. and V. Ambros, *An extensive class of small RNAs in Caenorhabditis elegans.* Science, 2001. **294**(5543): p. 862–4.

[23] Bushati, N.and S.M. Cohen, *microRNA functions.* Annu Rev Cell Dev Biol, 2007. **23**: p. 175–205.

[24] Jiu, S., X. Zhu, J. Wang, C. Zhang, Q. Mu, C. Wang, J. Fang, *Genome-wide mapping and analysis of grapevine microRNAs and their potential target genes.* The Plant Genome, 2015. **8**: p. 1–16.

[25] Lewis, B.P., et al., *Prediction of mammalian microRNA targets.* Cell, 2003. **115**(7): p. 787–98.

[26] Liu, B., J. Li, and M.J. Cairns, *Identifying miRNAs, targets and functions.* Brief Bioinform, 2014. **15**(1): p. 1–19.

[27] Ha, M. and V.N. Kim, *Regulation of microRNA biogenesis.* Nat Rev Mol Cell Biol, 2014. **15**(8): p. 509–24.

[28] Westholm, J.O. and E.C. Lai, *Mirtrons: microRNA biogenesis via splicing.* Biochimie, 2011. **93**(11): p. 1897–904.

[29] Abdelfattah, A.M., C. Park, and M.Y. Choi, *Update on non-canonical microRNAs.* Biomol Concepts, 2014. **5**(4): p. 275–87.

[30] Krol, J., I. Loedige, and W. Filipowicz, *The widespread regulation of microRNA biogenesis, function and decay.* Nat Rev Genet, 2010. **11**(9): p. 597–610.

[31] Havens, M.A., et al., *Biogenesis of mammalian microRNAs by a non-canonical processing pathway.* Nucleic Acids Res, 2012. **40**(10): p. 4626–40.

[32] Ameres, S.L. and P.D. Zamore, *Diversifying microRNA sequence and function.* Nat Rev Mol Cell Biol, 2013. **14**(8): p. 475–88.

[33] Stenvang, J., et al., *Inhibition of microRNA function by antimiR oligonucleotides.* Silence, 2012. **3**(1): p. 1.

[34] Miao, C.G., et al., *Critical roles of microRNAs in the pathogenesis of systemic sclerosis: New advances, challenges and potential directions.* Int Immunopharmacol, 2015. **28**(1): p. 626–33.

[35] Lai, E.C., *miRNAs: whys and wherefores of miRNA-mediated regulation.* Curr Biol, 2005. **15**(12): p. R458–60.

[36] Chen, X.M., et al., *Role of Micro RNAs in the Pathogenesis of Rheumatoid Arthritis: Novel Perspectives Based on Review of the Literature.* Medicine (Baltimore), 2015. **94**(31): p. e1326.

[37] Sharma, A.R., et al., *miRNA-regulated key components of cytokine signaling pathways and inflammation in rheumatoid arthritis.* Med Res Rev, 2016. **36**(3): p. 425–39.

[38] Luo, X., et al., *Evidence for microRNA-mediated regulation in rheumatic diseases.* Ann Rheum Dis, 2010. **69 Suppl 1**: p. i30–36.

[39] Dai, R. and S.A. Ahmed, *MicroRNA, a new paradigm for understanding immunoregulation, inflammation, and autoimmune diseases.* Transl Res, 2011. **157**(4): p. 163–79.

[40] Filipowicz, W., S.N. Bhattacharyya, and N. Sonenberg, *Mechanisms of post-transcriptional regulation by microRNAs: Are the answers in sight?* Nat Rev Genet, 2008. **9**(2): p. 102–14.

[41] Doench, J.G. and P.A. Sharp, *Specificity of microRNA target selection in translational repression.* Genes Dev, 2004. **18**(5): p. 504–11.

[42] Alipoor, S.D., et al., *The roles of miRNAs as potential biomarkers in lung diseases.* Eur J Pharmacol, 2016. **791**: p. 395–404.

[43] Nilsen, T.W., *Mechanisms of microRNA-mediated gene regulation in animal cells.* Trends Genet, 2007. **23**(5): p. 243–9.

[44] Vidigal, J.A. and A. Ventura, *The biological functions of miRNAs: lessons from in vivo studies.* Trends Cell Biol, 2015. **25**(3): p. 137–47.

[45] Pauley, K.M., S. Cha, and E.K. Chan, *MicroRNA in autoimmunity and autoimmune diseases.* J Autoimmun, 2009. **32**(3–4): p. 189–94.

[46] O'Connell, R.M., D.S. Rao, and D. Baltimore, *microRNA regulation of inflammatory responses.* Annu Rev Immunol, 2012. **30**: p. 295–312.

[47] Kawai, T. and S. Akira, *Toll-like receptors and their crosstalk with other innate receptors in infection and immunity.* Immunity, 2011. **34**(5): p. 637–50.

[48] Roach, J.C., et al., *The evolution of vertebrate Toll-like receptors.* Proc Natl Acad Sci U S A, 2005. **102**(27): p. 9577–82.

[49] Takeda, K. and S. Akira, *Toll-like receptors in innate immunity.* Int Immunol, 2005. **17**(1): p. 1–14.

[50] Chen, J.Q., P. Szodoray, and M. Zeher, *Toll-Like Receptor Pathways in Autoimmune Diseases.* Clin Rev Allergy Immunol, 2016. **50**(1): p. 1–17.

[51] Taganov, K.D., et al., *NF-kappaB-dependent induction of microRNA miR-146, an inhibitor targeted to signaling proteins of innate immune responses.* Proc Natl Acad Sci U S A, 2006. **103**(33): p. 12481–6.

[52] Hou, J., et al., *MicroRNA-146a feedback inhibits RIG-I-dependent Type I IFN production in macrophages by targeting TRAF6, IRAK1, and IRAK2.* J Immunol, 2009. **183**(3): p. 2150–8.

[53] Tili, E., et al., *Modulation of miR-155 and miR-125b levels following lipopolysaccharide/TNF-alpha stimulation and their possible roles in regulating the response to endotoxin shock.* J Immunol, 2007. **179**(8): p. 5082–9.

[54] Liu, G., et al., *miR-147, a microRNA that is induced upon Toll-like receptor stimulation, regulates murine macrophage inflammatory responses.* Proc Natl Acad Sci U S A, 2009. **106**(37): p. 15819–24.

[55] Au, K.Y., et al., *MiR-1303 regulates mycobacteria induced autophagy by targeting Atg2B.* PLoS One, 2016. **11**(1): p. e0146770.

[56] Husakova, M., *MicroRNAs in the key events of systemic lupus erythematosus pathogenesis.* Biomed Pap Med Fac Univ Palacky Olomouc Czech Repub, 2016. **160**(3): p. 327–42.

[57] de Yebenes, V.G., et al., *miR-181b negatively regulates activation-induced cytidine deaminase in B cells.* J Exp Med, 2008. **205**(10): p. 2199–206.

[58] Gonzalez-Martin, A., et al., *The microRNA miR-148a functions as a critical regulator of B cell tolerance and autoimmunity.* Nat Immunol, 2016. **17**(4): p. 433–40.

[59] Cobb, B.S., et al., *T cell lineage choice and differentiation in the absence of the RNase III enzyme Dicer.* J Exp Med, 2005. **201**(9): p. 1367–73.

[60] Koralov, S.B., et al., *Dicer ablation affects antibody diversity and cell survival in the B lymphocyte lineage.* Cell, 2008. **132**(5): p. 860–74.

[61] Honardoost, M.A., et al., *miR-326 and miR-26a, two potential markers for diagnosis of relapse and remission phases in patient with relapsing-remitting multiple sclerosis.* Gene, 2014. **544**(2): p. 128–33.

[62] Ceppi, M., et al., *MicroRNA-155 modulates the interleukin-1 signaling pathway in activated human monocyte-derived dendritic cells.* Proc Natl Acad Sci U S A, 2009. **106**(8): p. 2735–40.

[63] O'Connell, R.M., et al., *MicroRNA-155 promotes autoimmune inflammation by enhancing inflammatory T cell development.* Immunity, 2010. **33**(4): p. 607–19.

[64] Lu, L.F., et al., *Function of miR-146a in controlling Treg cell-mediated regulation of Th1 responses.* Cell, 2010. **142**(6): p. 914–29.

[65] Alamanos, Y. and A.A. Drosos, *Epidemiology of adult rheumatoid arthritis.* Autoimmun Rev, 2005. **4**(3): p. 130–6.

[66] Ahlmen, M., et al., *Influence of gender on assessments of disease activity and function in early rheumatoid arthritis in relation to radiographic joint damage.* Ann Rheum Dis, 2010. **69**(1): p. 230–3.

[67] Areskoug-Josefsson, K. and U. Oberg, *A literature review of the sexual health of women with rheumatoid arthritis.* Musculoskeletal Care, 2009. **7**(4): p. 219–26.

[68] Rossini, M., et al., *Prevalence and incidence of rheumatoid arthritis in Italy.* Rheumatol Int, 2014. **34**(5): p. 659–64.

[69] Smolen, J.S., et al., *Treating rheumatoid arthritis to target: 2014 update of the recommendations of an international task force.* Ann Rheum Dis, 2016. **75**(1): p. 3–15.

[70] Uhlig, T., R.H. Moe, and T.K. Kvien, *The burden of disease in rheumatoid arthritis.* Pharmacoeconomics, 2014. **32**(9): p. 841–51.

[71] Vojdani, A., *A potential link between environmental triggers and autoimmunity.* Autoimmune Dis, 2014. **2014**: p. 437231.

[72] Iborra, M., et al., *MicroRNAs in autoimmunity and inflammatory bowel disease: crucial regulators in immune response.* Autoimmun Rev, 2012. **11**(5): p. 305–14.

[73] Jimenez, S.A. and S. Piera-Velazquez, *Potential role of human-specific genes, human-specific microRNAs and human-specific non-coding regulatory RNAs in the pathogenesis of systemic sclerosis and Sjogren's syndrome.* Autoimmun Rev, 2013. **12**(11): p. 1046–51.

[74] Thamilarasan, M., et al., *MicroRNAs in multiple sclerosis and experimental autoimmune encephalomyelitis.* Autoimmun Rev, 2012. **11**(3): p. 174–9.

[75] Singh, R.P., et al., *The role of miRNA in inflammation and autoimmunity.* Autoimmun Rev, 2013. **12**(12): p. 1160–5.

[76] Chatzikyriakidou, A., et al., *miRNAs and related polymorphisms in rheumatoid arthritis susceptibility.* Autoimmun Rev, 2012. **11**(9): p. 636–41.

[77] Salehi, E., et al., *MicroRNAs in rheumatoid arthritis.* Clin Rheumatol, 2015. **34**(4): p. 615–28.

[78] Stanczyk, J., et al., *Altered expression of microRNA in synovial fibroblasts and synovial tissue in rheumatoid arthritis.* Arthritis Rheum, 2008. **58**(4): p. 1001–9.

[79] Wittmann, J. and H.M. Jack, *microRNAs in rheumatoid arthritis: midget RNAs with a giant impact.* Ann Rheum Dis, 2011. **70 Suppl 1**: p. i92–6.

[80] Shibuya, H., et al., *Overexpression of microRNA-223 in rheumatoid arthritis synovium controls osteoclast differentiation.* Mod Rheumatol, 2013. **23**(4): p. 674–85.

[81] Nakasa, T., et al., *Expression of microRNA-146 in rheumatoid arthritis synovial tissue.* Arthritis Rheum, 2008. **58**(5): p. 1284–92.

[82] Niimoto, T., et al., *MicroRNA-146a expresses in interleukin-17 producing T cells in rheumatoid arthritis patients.* BMC Musculoskelet Disord, 2010. **11**: p. 209.

[83] Zhu, S., et al., *The microRNA miR-23b suppresses IL-17-associated autoimmune inflammation by targeting TAB2, TAB3 and IKK-alpha.* Nat Med, 2012. **18**(7): p. 1077–86.

[84] Xu, K., et al., *Reduced apoptosis correlates with enhanced autophagy in synovial tissues of rheumatoid arthritis.* Inflamm Res, 2013. **62**(2): p. 229–37.

[85] Lin, J., et al., *A novel p53/microRNA-22/Cyr61 axis in synovial cells regulates inflammation in rheumatoid arthritis.* Arthritis Rheumatol, 2014. **66**(1): p. 49–59.

[86] Murata, K., et al., *Plasma and synovial fluid microRNAs as potential biomarkers of rheumatoid arthritis and osteoarthritis.* Arthritis Res Ther, 2010. **12**(3): p. R86.

[87] Churov, A.V., E.K. Oleinik, and M. Knip, *MicroRNAs in rheumatoid arthritis: altered expression and diagnostic potential.* Autoimmun Rev, 2015. **14**(11): p. 1029–37.

[88] Nakamachi, Y., et al., *MicroRNA-124a is a key regulator of proliferation and monocyte chemoattractant protein 1 secretion in fibroblast-like synoviocytes from patients with rheumatoid arthritis.* Arthritis Rheum, 2009. **60**(5): p. 1294–304.

[89] Niederer, F., et al., *Down-regulation of microRNA-34a* in rheumatoid arthritis synovial fibroblasts promotes apoptosis resistance.* Arthritis Rheum, 2012. **64**(6): p. 1771–9.

[90] Pandis, I., et al., *Identification of microRNA-221/222 and microRNA-323-3p association with rheumatoid arthritis via predictions using the human tumour necrosis factor transgenic mouse model.* Ann Rheum Dis, 2012. **71**(10): p. 1716–23.

[91] Stanczyk, J., et al., *Altered expression of microRNA-203 in rheumatoid arthritis synovial fibroblasts and its role in fibroblast activation.* Arthritis Rheum, 2011. **63**(2): p. 373–81.

[92] Miao, C.G., et al., *MicroRNA-152 modulates the canonical Wnt pathway activation by targeting DNA methyltransferase 1 in arthritic rat model.* Biochimie, 2014. **106**: p. 149–56.

[93] Miao, C.G., et al., *miR-375 regulates the canonical Wnt pathway through FZD8 silencing in arthritis synovial fibroblasts.* Immunol Lett, 2015. **164**(1): p. 1–10.

[94] Kurowska-Stolarska, M., et al., *MicroRNA-155 as a proinflammatory regulator in clinical and experimental arthritis.* Proc Natl Acad Sci U S A, 2011. **108**(27): p. 11193–8.

[95] Duroux-Richard, I., et al., *Circulating miRNA-125b is a potential biomarker predicting response to rituximab in rheumatoid arthritis.* Mediators Inflamm, 2014. **2014**: p. 342524.

[96] Mookherjee, N. and H.S. El-Gabalawy, *High degree of correlation between whole blood and PBMC expression levels of miR-155 and miR-146a in healthy controls and rheumatoid arthritis patients.* J Immunol Methods, 2013. **400-401**: p. 106–10.

[97] Pauley, K.M., et al., *Upregulated miR-146a expression in peripheral blood mononuclear cells from rheumatoid arthritis patients.* Arthritis Res Ther, 2008. **10**(4): p. R101.

[98] Filkova, M., et al., *Association of circulating miR-223 and miR-16 with disease activity in patients with early rheumatoid arthritis.* Ann Rheum Dis, 2014. **73**(10): p. 1898–904.

[99] Wang, H., et al., *Circulating microRNAs as candidate biomarkers in patients with systemic lupus erythematosus.* Transl Res, 2012. **160**(3): p. 198–206.

[100] Murata, K., et al., *Comprehensive microRNA analysis identifies miR-24 and miR-125a-5p as plasma biomarkers for rheumatoid arthritis.* PLoS One, 2013. **8**(7): p. e69118.

[101] Nagata, Y., et al., *Induction of apoptosis in the synovium of mice with autoantibody-mediated arthritis by the intraarticular injection of double-stranded MicroRNA-15a.* Arthritis Rheum, 2009. **60**(9): p. 2677–83.

[102] Philippe, L., et al., *The miR-17 approximately 92 cluster: A key player in the control of inflammation during rheumatoid arthritis.* Front Immunol, 2013. **4**: p. 70.

[103] Trenkmann, M., et al., *Tumor necrosis factor alpha-induced microRNA-18a activates rheumatoid arthritis synovial fibroblasts through a feedback loop in NF-kappaB signaling.* Arthritis Rheum, 2013. **65**(4): p. 916–27.

[104] Dong, L., et al., *Decreased expression of microRNA-21 correlates with the imbalance of Th17 and Treg cells in patients with rheumatoid arthritis.* J Cell Mol Med, 2014. **18**(11): p. 2213–24.

[105] Tardif, G., et al., *Regulation of the IGFBP-5 and MMP-13 genes by the microRNAs miR-140 and miR-27a in human osteoarthritic chondrocytes.* BMC Musculoskelet Disord, 2009. **10**: p. 148.

[106] Akhtar, N., et al., *MicroRNA-27b regulates the expression of matrix metalloproteinase 13 in human osteoarthritis chondrocytes.* Arthritis Rheum, 2010. **62**(5): p. 1361–71.

[107] Alsaleh, G., et al., *MiR-30a-3p negatively regulates BAFF synthesis in systemic sclerosis and rheumatoid arthritis fibroblasts.* PLoS One, 2014. **9**(10): p. e111266.

[108] Kim, S.W., et al., *MicroRNAs miR-125a and miR-125b constitutively activate the NF-kappaB pathway by targeting the tumor necrosis factor alpha-induced protein 3 (TNFAIP3, A20).* Proc Natl Acad Sci U S A, 2012. **109**(20): p. 7865–70.

[109] Hruskova, V., et al., *MicroRNA-125b: association with disease activity and the treatment response of patients with early rheumatoid arthritis.* Arthritis Res Ther, 2016. **18**(1): p. 124.

[110] Gao, J., et al., *microRNA-126 targeting PIK3R2 promotes rheumatoid arthritis synovial fibroblasts proliferation and resistance to apoptosis by regulating PI3K/AKT pathway.* Exp Mol Pathol, 2016. **100**(1): p. 192–8.

[111] O'Neill, L.A., *Boosting the brain's ability to block inflammation via microRNA-132.* Immunity, 2009. **31**(6): p. 854–5.

[112] Dong, S., et al., *MicroRNAs regulate osteogenesis and chondrogenesis.* Biochem Biophys Res Commun, 2012. **418**(4): p. 587–91.

[113] Yamasaki, K., et al., *Expression of microRNA-146a in osteoarthritis cartilage.* Arthritis Rheum, 2009. **60**(4): p. 1035–41.

[114] Li, J., et al., *Altered microRNA expression profile with miR-146a upregulation in CD4+ T cells from patients with rheumatoid arthritis.* Arthritis Res Ther, 2010. **12**(3): p. R81.

[115] Abou-Zeid, A., M. Saad, and E. Soliman, *MicroRNA 146a expression in rheumatoid arthritis: association with tumor necrosis factor-alpha and disease activity.* Genet Test Mol Biomarkers, 2011. **15**(11): p. 807–12.

[116] Zhou, Q., et al., *Decreased expression of miR-146a and miR-155 contributes to an abnormal Treg phenotype in patients with rheumatoid arthritis.* Ann Rheum Dis, 2015. **74**(6): p. 1265–74.

[117] Guo, M., et al., *miR-146a in PBMCs modulates Th1 function in patients with acute coronary syndrome.* Immunol Cell Biol, 2010. **88**(5): p. 555–64.

[118] Swingler, T.E., et al., *The expression and function of microRNAs in chondrogenesis and osteoarthritis.* Arthritis Rheum, 2012. **64**(6): p. 1909–19.

[119] Yang, S. and Y. Yang, *Downregulation of microRNA221 decreases migration and invasion in fibroblastlike synoviocytes in rheumatoid arthritis.* Mol Med Rep, 2015. **12**(2): p. 2395–401.

[120] Lu, M.C., et al., *Increased miR-223 expression in T cells from patients with rheumatoid arthritis leads to decreased insulin-like growth factor-1-mediated interleukin-10 production.* Clin Exp Immunol, 2014. **177**(3): p. 641–51.

[121] Fulci, V., et al., *miR-223 is overexpressed in T-lymphocytes of patients affected by rheumatoid arthritis.* Hum Immunol, 2010. **71**(2): p. 206–11.

[122] Murata, K., et al., *MicroRNA-451 down-regulates neutrophil chemotaxis via p38 MAPK.* Arthritis Rheumatol, 2014. **66**(3): p. 549–59.

[123] Krintel, S.B., et al., *Prediction of treatment response to adalimumab: a double-blind placebo-controlled study of circulating microRNA in patients with early rheumatoid arthritis.* Pharmacogenomics J, 2016. **16**(2): p. 141–6.

[124] Jiang, S., T.E. Hinchliffe, and T. Wu, *Biomarkers of an autoimmune skin disease—Psoriasis.* Genomics Proteomics Bioinformatics, 2015. **13**(4): p. 224–33.

[125] Ichihara, A., et al., *Increased serum levels of miR-1266 in patients with psoriasis vulgaris.* Eur J Dermatol, 2012. **22**(1): p. 68–71.

[126] Lovendorf, M.B., et al., *MicroRNA-223 and miR-143 are important systemic biomarkers for disease activity in psoriasis.* J Dermatol Sci, 2014. **75**(2): p. 133–9.

[127] Chandra, A., et al., *Genetic and epigenetic basis of psoriasis pathogenesis.* Mol Immunol, 2015. **64**(2): p. 313–23.

[128] Joyce, C.E., et al., *Deep sequencing of small RNAs from human skin reveals major alterations in the psoriasis miRNAome.* Hum Mol Genet, 2011. **20**(20): p. 4025–40.

[129] Dai, Y., et al., *Microarray analysis of microRNA expression in peripheral blood cells of systemic lupus erythematosus patients.* Lupus, 2007. **16**(12): p. 939–46.

[130] Dai, Y., et al., *Comprehensive analysis of microRNA expression patterns in renal biopsies of lupus nephritis patients.* Rheumatol Int, 2009. **29**(7): p. 749–54.

[131] Tang, Y., et al., *MicroRNA-146A contributes to abnormal activation of the type I interferon pathway in human lupus by targeting the key signaling proteins.* Arthritis Rheum, 2009. **60**(4): p. 1065–75.

[132] Otaegui, D., et al., *Differential micro RNA expression in PBMC from multiple sclerosis patients.* PLoS One, 2009. **4**(7): p. e6309.

[133] Brown, K.D., E. Claudio, and U. Siebenlist, *The roles of the classical and alternative nuclear factor-kappaB pathways: potential implications for autoimmunity and rheumatoid arthritis.* Arthritis Res Ther, 2008. **10**(4): p. 212.

Section 2

Immune Response in Rheumatoid Arthritis

Chapter 3

Cytokines in Rheumatoid Arthritis (RA)

Selim Nalbant and Ahmet Merih Birlik

Additional information is available at the end of the chapter

http://dx.doi.org/10.5772/65893

Abstract

Cytokines are cell molecules that are secreted by immune cells and aid cell to cell communication in immune responses and stimulate the movement of cells towards sites of inflammation, infection and trauma. So, the cytokines are the main part of the immune network to provide the communication in rheumatoid arthritis (RA) too. In RA, cytokines may be classified into four groups: pro-inflammatory cytokines, inflammatory cytokines in joints, anti-inflammatory cytokines and natural cytokine antagonists. After the initial stimuli have occurred, cytokines play a role in communication between the parts of immune system in every step of the pathophysiology process of RA. The differentiation of narve T cells into Th17 cells results in inflammation (synovitis) in joints. B cells further the pathogenic process through antigen presentation and autoantibody and cytokine production. The release of cytokines, especially tumor necrosis factor (TNF)-α, interleukin (IL)-6 and IL-1, causes synovial inflammation. In addition to their articular effects, pro-inflammatory cytokines promote the development of systemic effects (anemia, cardiovascular disease, fatigue and depression). So, cytokines are the main molecules contributing to all facets of the disease.

Keywords: cytokines, effector cells, rheumatoid arthritis, anti-cytokine treatment

1. Cytokine and rheumatoid arthritis

Rheumatoid arthritis (RA) is a progressive inflammatory disease, which is characterized by symmetrical polyarthritis. As an inflammatory disease, RA is characterized by increased levels in pro-inflammatory cytokines. In this complex cytokine environment, apart from arthritis, systemic manifestations also occur. Genetic and environmental factors are contributory to this complex nature of RA process. T cells, B cells and their cytokines play key roles in the pathophysiology of RA. Today's modern RA treatment basically targets these cytokines. While we do this, we are generally treat the *"normal and abnormal cytokine response"* at the same time, because we do not know the main etiology of this abnormal cytokine response. To better manage RA, we should understand the role of cytokines and the relation between the effector cells [1–6].

The term "**cytokine**" is derived from a combination of two Greek words–"cyto" **meaning** cell and "kine" **meaning** move. **Cytokines** are cell molecules that are secreted by immune cells and aid cell to cell communication in cases of inflammation, infection and injury. So, the cytokines are vital part of the immune network to provide communication [7].

2. What is the origin of this complex cytokine response?

RA is an autoimmune disease. The term autoimmunity usually means a lot information that defines ***the way*** but not ***the origin of the process***, and this stands for RA too. On the other hand, autoimmunity also means autoantibody production. In RA, there are two autoantibodies, rheumatoid factor and anti-cyclic citrullinated peptide antibodies, which contribute to inflammation. In the end, chronic inflammatory arthritis and the organ damage occur [8, 9].

The very early events of RA pathogenesis get into motion by breaking T-cell and/or B-cell tolerance and/or ignorance. However, this mechanism was poorly defined. After, shaping of this autoimmune background, some subsequent events intervene to perpetuate the process of synovial inflammation. What directs this process to the joints is unknown and it probably includes biomechanical factors, neuro-immuno-endocrinological interactions and altered articular microvascular microenvironment. Several factors have been proposed to have an association with the susceptibility and severity of rheumatoid arthritis [1–10].

These factors are as follows:

(1) Genetic loci:

- HLA-DR4 alleles
- *PTPN22* (protein tyrosine phosphatase, nonreceptor type 22)
- *PADI4* (peptidyl arginine deiminase, type IV)
- *CTLA4* (cytotoxic T-lymphocyte antigen 4)
- FcγRs (Fc receptors for IgG)
- Various cytokine and cytokine-receptor loci.

(2) Environmental factors (smoking, stress, hormonal factors, etc.)

(3) Infectious organisms
The earliest event in RA pathogenesis perhaps is activation of the innate immune response. In this first step, cytokines play a role in communication between the parts of immune system. In second step, antigen-presenting cells present arthritis-associated antigens to T cells. This step is the starting point of the cytokine effect, which augments the inflammation and

stimulate the other systems (such as lipid mediators, nitric oxide, RANKL-RANK signaling, etc.) that cause joint destruction and the organ damage [11–13].

3. How can we classify this cytokine network in RA

Actually to make classification of cytokines for rheumatoid arthritis is not feasible. Because many of them have some pleotropic effect at the same time. However, we may basically, classify cytokines four groups in the pathogenesis of rheumatoid arthritis. Actually, this classification is not a real one, it is just for the establishment of understanding the whole mechanism [10] (**Table 1**).

1. Pro-inflammatory cytokines: IL-1 and TNF-alpha cytokine role in

IL-1

- Increased synovial fibroblast cytokine, chemokine, MMP and PG release
- Increased monocyte cytokine, reactive oxygen intermediate and PG release
- Osteoclast activation
- Endothelial cell adhesion molecule expression
- Acute-phase protein production
- Cardiovascular disease promotion
- HPA axis dysregulation (fatigue and depression) [2, 14, 15]

TNF-alpha

- Increased monocyte activation, cytokine release, prostaglandin release
- T-cell clonal regulation
- Increased endothelial cell adhesion molecule expression, cytokine release
- Acute-phase protein production and fatigue-depression [2, 16]

2. Inflammatory cytokines in joints: IL-1 and TNF-alpha, IL-6, IL-15, IL-16, IL-17, IL-18, IFN-gamma, granulocyte macrophage-colony stimulating factor

IL 6

- Osteoclast and B-cell activation
- T-cell proliferation and differentiation
- Acute-phase protein and hepcidin (anemia) production [17, 18]

IL-15

- Structural similarities to IL-2,4 produced primarily by macrophages
- Regulation of synovial inflammation [19–21]

IL-16

- Suppression of IFN-γ, TNF-α and IL-1β expression
- Anti-inflammatory effect by regulation of Tregs [22]

IL-17

- Increase local chemokine production
- Augmentation of immune response (increase IL-6 production)
- Cartilage damage
- Promotes the effect of IL-1b, TNF-a and IFN-g [20, 23, 24]

IL-18

- Increase the production of pro-inflammatory cytokines, chemokines, adhesion molecules and RANKL which are the main molecules of joint destruction
- Increase the production of fibroblast-like synoviocytes and chondrocytes [25, 26]

IL-21

- Activate TH17 cells
- Induces osteoclastogenesis
- Plasma levels shows correlation with DAS28 [2]

IFN-gamma

- Immune modulation (both protection and activation) [27, 28]

Granulocyte macrophage-colony stimulating factor (GM-CSF)

- Promotes existing RA [29]

3. Anti-inflammatory cytokines

IL-10

- Inhibit Th1 cell activity by suppressing IFN-γ expression
- Direct inhibitory effect on the macrophage activity in the synovium
- Elevated levels in the synovial fluid
- Dominant suppressive cytokine effect
- Protection against cartilage destruction combination with IL-4 [2, 7]

IL-4

- Increased level in synovial fluid during only synovial inflammation
- Preventing collagen type I breakdown in RA [30–33]

IL-13

- Synergistic or inhibitory roles during the arthritis with IL-10, IL-21R, galectin-3 and TGFβ [34]

IL-20

- Regulates osteoclast differentiation [35]

4-Natural cytokine antagonists

IL-1 receptor antagonist (IL-1ra)

- Low levels of IL-1 receptor antagonist (IL-1ra) causes erosive disease in patients and [36]

http://dx.doi.org/10.5772/65893

Soluble type 2 IL-1 receptor	
• Cause competitive inhibition by binding interleukin-1α (IL1A), interleukin-1β (IL1B) and interleukin 1 receptor antagonist (IL1Ra), and acts as a pseudo receptor activity that inhibits the activity of its ligands [37, 38]	
Soluble TNF receptor (sTNF-RI)	
• It is not well-known; possible effect is to cause cleavage of TNF alpha [39]	
IL-18 binding protein	
• Protect against the joint destructive effect by binding IL-18 in RA [40]	

Table 1. Actions of cytokines that play major roles in RA pathobiology.

3.1. Pro-inflammatory cytokines

Interleukin (IL)-1 and tumor necrosis factor (TNF)-alpha are the main pro-inflammatory cytokines involved in RA. The influx and/or local activation of mononuclear cells and the formation of new blood vessels are main findings in synovial membrane. Differentiation of naive T cells into Th17 cells contributes to synovitis. B cells further the pathogenic process through antigen presentation and autoantibody and cytokine production. Enzymes secreted by synoviocytes and chondrocytes degrade cartilage. The release of cytokines, especially TNF-alpha and IL-1, have multiple detrimental effects on cartilage and bone. Pro-inflammatory cytokines act locally but also have systemic effects, such as production of acute-phase proteins, anemia of chronic disease, cardiovascular disease, osteoporosis, etc. [1–7, 11, 12].

3.2. Inflammatory cytokines in joints

These cytokines are basically cytokine found in higher levels in the joints of patients with RA than in the serum. Most are pro-inflammatory cytokines. They cause mostly local joint destruction and also systemic effects of the disease and include IL-1, TNF-alpha, IL-6, IL-15, IL-16, IL-17, IL-18, interferon (IFN)-γ, granulocyte macrophage-colony stimulating factor) [10–12].

3.3. Anti-inflammatory cytokines: (IL-4, IL-10, IL-11, IL-13 and IL-20)

In case of an inflammatory state, such as RA, the immune system utilizes anti-inflammatory cytokines to restrict the inflammatory reaction. In RA synovitis, there is an imbalance between pro-inflammatory and anti-inflammatory cytokines due to insufficient local concentrations of anti-inflammatory cytokines, IL-10, IL-11 and IL-13 to mediate counter-regulatory activity against the dominant pro-inflammatory cytokines. This is almost valid for the T-cell-derived cytokines, which are IL-2 and IL-4. They are also absent, which may impair Treg-cell generation and favor TH1-cell or TH17-cell immune responses [1, 2, 10].

3.4. Natural cytokine antagonists

Immune system is the most complex system, which has a self-limiting or self-controlling mechanism. The known molecules for this purpose are IL-1 receptor antagonist (IL-1ra), soluble type 2 IL-1 receptor, soluble TNF receptor (sTNF-RI) and IL-18 binding protein. However, current information about them is not entirely known. It is suggested that TNFR1 and the type II IL-1R have a regulatory role in sequestering soluble TNF and IL-1 away from their cell-bound receptors. Their detected levels in synovial tissues and fluid are insufficient to counteract the inflammatory cytokines and bring cytokine homeostasis. We currently use these natural anti-inflammatory molecules for therapeutic reasons [1–6].

4. Conclusion

As a result, cytokine effects do not occur with a single cytokine signalling cascade. There are many factors effecting the cytokine response. These are not only to control the equilibrium between inflammatory and anti-inflammatory cytokines but also the pleotropic and individual effects of cytokines. Here, we describe the topics of cytokine network only. It will be crucial to select cytokine targets based not on one single inflammatory pathway but rather on a biosystematic approach to pathogenesis. Implicit in this will be the recognition of pivotal checkpoints that facilitate the progression from autoimmunity to chronic inflammation [1, 11–13].

As it was seen, cytokines are the main molecules at all these stages. However, they are not only the origin of the all cascade but also the last point which is occurring the damage. So, this fact makes the cytokine as a target molecule to treat.

Author details

Selim Nalbant[1,]* and Ahmet Merih Birlik[2]

*Address all correspondence to: nalbantselim@hotmail.com

1 Department of Internal Medicine, Medical Faculty of Maltepe University, Istanbul, Turkey

2 Department of Immunology and Rheumatology of Medical School of Dokuz Eylul Universty, Izmir, Turkey

References

[1] Feldmann, M., Brennan, F. M. & Maini, R. N. Rheumatoid arthritis. Cell 1996; **85**: 307–310.

[2] Feldmann, M., Brennan, F. M. & Maini, R. N. Role of cytokines in rheumatoid arthritis. Annu. Rev. Immunol. 1996; **14**: 397–440.

[3] Firestein, G. S. Evolving concepts of rheumatoid arthritis. Nature 2003; **423**: 356–361.

[4] McInnes, I. B. & Liew, F. Y. Cytokine networks—towards new therapies for rheumatoid arthritis. Nat. Clin. Pract. Rheumatol 2005; **1**: 31–39.

[5] Venkatesha, S. H., Dudics, S., Acharya, B. & Kamal D. Moudgil. Cytokine-modulating strategies and newer cytokine targets for arthritis therapy. Int. J. Mol. Sci. 2015; **16**: 887–906.

[6] Ponchel, F., Goëb, V., Parmar, R., El-Sherbiny, Y., Boissinot, M., El Jawhari, J., Burska, A., Vital, E. M., Harrison, S., Conaghan, P. G., Hensor, E & Emery, P. An immunological biomarker to predict MTX response in early RA. Ann. Rheum. Dis. 2014; **73**(11): 2047–2053.

[7] Kasama, T., Isozaki, T., Takahashi, R. & Miwa, Y. Clinical effects of tocilizumab on cytokines and immunological factors in patients with rheumatoid arthritis. Int. Immunopharmacol. 2016; **35**: 301–306.

[8] Burmester, G. R. et al. Emerging cell and cytokine targets in rheumatoid arthritis. Nat. Rev. Rheumatol. 2014; **10**: 77–88.

[9] van der Helm-van Mil, A. H., Wesoly, J. Z. & Huizinga, T. W. Understanding the genetic contribution to rheumatoid arthritis. Curr. Opin. Rheumatol. 2005; **17**: 299–304.

[10] Choy, E. Understanding the dynamics: pathways involved in the pathogenesis of rheumatoid arthritis. Rheumatology 2012; **51**: 3–11.

[11] Jimenez-Boj, E. et al. Interaction between synovial inflammatory tissue and bone marrow in rheumatoid arthritis. J. Immunol. 2005; **175**: 2579–2588.

[12] Chabaud, M. et al. Human interleukin-17: a T cell-derived proinflammatory cytokine produced by the rheumatoid synovium. Arthritis Rheum. 1999; **42**: 963–970.

[13] Joosten, L. A. et al. IL-32, a proinflammatory cytokine in rheumatoid arthritis. Proc. Natl. Acad. Sci. 2006; **103**: 3298–3303.

[14] Dayer, J. M. & Bresnihan, B. Targeting interleukin-1 in the treatment of rheumatoid arthritis. Arthritis Rheum. 2002; **46**: 574–578.

[15] Horai, R. et al. Development of chronic inflammatory arthropathy resembling rheumatoid arthritis in interleukin 1 receptor antagonist-deficient mice. J. Exp. Med. 2000; **191**: 313–320.

[16] Redlich, K. et al. Osteoclasts are essential for TNF-α-mediated joint destruction. J. Clin. Invest. 2002; **110**: 1419–1427.

[17] Nishimoto, N. & Kishimoto, T. Interleukin 6: from bench to bedside. Nat. Clin. Pract. Rheumatol. 2006; **2**: 619–626.

[18] Alonzi, T. et al. Interleukin 6 is required for the development of collagen-induced arthritis. J. Exp. Med. 1998; **187**: 461–468.

[19] McInnes, I. B., Leung, B. P., Sturrock, R. D., Field, M. & Liew, F. Y. Interleukin-15 mediates T celldependent regulation of tumor necrosis factor-α production in rheumatoid arthritis. Nat. Med. 1997;**3**: 189–195.

[20] Ferrari-Lacraz, S. et al. Targeting IL-15 receptor bearing cells with an antagonist mutant IL-15/Fc protein prevents disease development and progression in murine collagen-induced arthritis. J. Immunol. 2004; **173**: 5818–5826.

[21] Baslund, B. et al. Targeting interleukin-15 in patients with rheumatoid arthritis: a proof-of-concept study. Arthritis Rheum. 2005; **52**: 2686–2692.

[22] Suzuki, M., Konya, C., Goronzy, J. J. & Weyand, C. M. Inhibitory CD8+ T cells in autoimmune disease. Hum. Immunol. 2008; **69**(11): 781–789.

[23] Lubberts, E., Koenders, M. I. & van den Berg, W. B. The role of T-cell interleukin-17 in conducting destructive arthritis: lessons from animal models. Arthritis Res. Ther. 2005; **7**: 29–37.

[24] Weaver, C. T., Hatton, R. D., Mangan, P. R. & Harrington, L. E. IL-17 family cytokines and the expanding diversity of effector T cell lineages. Annu. Rev. Immunol. 2007; **25**: 821–852.

[25] Gracie, J. A. et al. A proinflammatory role for IL-18 in rheumatoid arthritis. J. Clin. Invest. 1999; **104**: 1393–1401.

[26] McInnes, I. B., Liew, F. Y. & Gracie, J. A. Interleukin-18: a therapeutic target in rheumatoid arthritis? Arthritis Res. Ther. 2004; **7**: 38–41.

[27] Manoury-Schwartz, B. et al. High susceptibility to collagen-induced arthritis in mice lacking IFN-γ receptors. J. Immunol. 1997; **158**: 5501–5506.

[28] Vermeire, K. et al. Accelerated collagen-induced arthritis in IFN-γ receptor-deficient mice. J. Immunol. 1997; **158**: 5507–5513.

[29] Di Franco, M., Gerardi, M. C., Lucchino, B. & Conti, F. Mavrilimumab: an evidence based review of its potential in the treatment of rheumatoid arthritis. Core Evid. 2014; 9: 41–48.

[30] Krabben A, Wilson AG, de Rooy DP, Zhernakova A, Brouwer E, Lindqvist E, Saxne T, Stoeken G, van Nies JA, Knevel R, Huizinga TW, Toes R, Gregersen PK, van der Helm-van Mil AH. Association of genetic variants in the IL4 and IL4R genes with the severity of joint damage in rheumatoid arthritis: a study in seven cohorts. Arthritis Rheum. 2013; **65**: 3051–7.

[31] Schulze-Koops, H. & Kalden, J. R. The balance of Th1/Th2 cytokines in rheumatoid arthritis. Best Pract. Res. Clin. Rheumatol. 2001; **15**: 677–691.

[32] Raza, K. et al. Early rheumatoid arthritis is characterized by a distinct and transientsy-novial fluid cytokine profile of T cell and stromal cell origin. Arthritis Res. Ther. 2005; **7**: R784–R795.

[33] Nalbant, S., Koc, B., Top, C., Kucukardali, Y., Baykal, Y., Danaci, M. & Kocer, I. Hypersensitivity vasculitis and cytokines. Rheumatol. Int. 2002; **22**(6): 244–248.

[34] Steven J. Van Dyken & Richard M. Locksley. Interleukin-4-and interleukin-13-mediated alternatively activated macrophages: roles in homeostasis and disease. Annu. Rev. Immunol. 2013; **31**: 317–343.

[35] Hsu, Y. H. & Chang, M. S. IL-20 in rheumatoid arthritis. Drug Discov Today. 2015; **19**. pii:S1359-6446(15)00312-8. doi:10.1016/j.drudis.2015.08.002 [Epub ahead of print]

[36] Cantagrel, A., Navaux, F., Loubet-Lescoulié, P., Nourhashemi, F., Enault, G., Abbal, M., Constantin, A., Laroche, M. & Maziéres, B. Interleukin-1β, interleukin-1 receptor antagonist, interleukin-4, and interleukin-10 gene polymorphisms: relationship to occurrence and severity of rheumatoid arthritis. Arthritis Rheum. 1999; **42**(6): 1093–1100.

[37] McMahan, C. J., Slack, J. L., Mosley, B., Cosman, D., Lupton, S. D., Brunton, L.L., Grubin, C. E., Wignall, J. M., Jenkins, N. A. & Brannan, C. I. A novel IL-1 receptor, cloned from B cells by mammalian expression, is expressed in many cell types. EMBO J. 1991; **10**(10): 2821–2832.

[38] Dripps, D. J., Verderber, E., Ng, R. K., Thompson, R. C. & Eisenberg, S. P. Interleukin-1 receptor antagonist binds to the type II interleukin-1 receptor on B cells and neutrophils. J. Biol. Chem. 1991; **266**(30): 20311–20315.

[39] Galvani, V. Soluble tumor necrosis factor receptor I (sTNFRI) as a prognostic factor in melanoma patients in Slovene population Article Pflügers Archiv. Eur. J. Physiol. 2000; **440**(5 Suppl): R61–R63.

[40] Bresnihan, B., Roux-Lombard, P., Murphy, E., Kane, D., FitzGerald, O., Dayer, J. M. Serum interleukin 18 and interleukin 18 binding protein in rheumatoid arthritis. Ann. Rheum. Dis. 2002; **61**: 726–729.

Chapter 4

BAFF System in Rheumatoid Arthritis: from Pathobiology to Therapeutic Targets

Codrina Ancuta, Cristina Pomirleanu,
Claudia Mihailov, Eugen Ancuta and Daniela Opris

Additional information is available at the end of the chapter

http://dx.doi.org/10.5772/66580

Abstract

Recent advances in understanding the multifaceted pathobiology of rheumatoid arthritis have highlighted the pivotal role and continuing crosstalk between activated immune cells, pro-inflammatory cytokines, and matrix-degrading mediators, promoting chronic inflammation as well as irreversible tissue damage within an autoimmune background. B cells are widely recognized as leading players in immune-mediated pathology based on their ability to produce not only different patterns of autoantibodies and driving cytokine synthesis but also as independent antigen-presenting cells and by modulating the specific activation of T cells. Overwhelming evidence emphasized the role of BAFF, a B-cell-activating factor, and BAFF receptors (TACI, BCMA, BAFF-R) in promoting B-cell homeostasis, proliferation, and survival under normal and autoimmune systemic disorders. We systematically reviewed data from literature focusing on BAFF, its homolog molecule APRIL, and BAFF-binding receptors biology, dysregulation of BAFF/BAFF receptor signaling in autoimmune settings, and current status of targeting BAFF/BAFF receptor pathway for rheumatoid arthritis.

Keywords: rheumatoid arthritis, autoimmunity, B-cell-activating factor (BAFF), BAFF-bounding receptors, BAFF antagonists

1. Introduction

Rheumatoid arthritis (RA) is a chronic immuno-inflammatory disease characterized by a multifaceted pathobiology, where a complex cytokine and cellular network contribute to excessive and extensive articular and systemic inflammatory events, accompanied by progressive tissue damage [1–4].

B cells are widely recognized as leading players in the mechanisms underlying the pathogenesis of RA based on their ability to produce not only different subsets of autoantibodies but also as independent antigen-presenting cells, cytokine synthesis, and modulators of T-cell activation. Moreover, their differentiation and survival are driven by positive feedback loops induced by cytokines, especially members belonging to the tumor necrosis factor (TNF) family [1–4].

Recent data highlighted the role of signaling crosstalk in B-lymphocytes, particularly of B-cell-activating factor (BAFF) and its receptors in early steps of the disease, advancing clinical development of BAFF antagonists for the treatment of RA [2–5]. Acting as an innate cytokine mediator, BAFF is known to modulate peripheral B- and T-cell homeostasis, promoting specific downstream signaling events through three different types of receptors [2, 4, 5].

Abnormal BAFF/BAFF receptor-signaling pathways were reported in several autoimmune disorders including systemic lupus erythematosus, Sjogren's syndrome, ANCA-associated vasculitis, and RA [2, 4, 5]. Of interest, elevated BAFF levels were detected in synovial fluid, serum, and saliva in very early stages of RA, suggesting its involvement in cell-cell interactions network in the synovial microenvironment, as well as B-cell activation and the development of autoreactive B cells [2–4]. Furthermore, the overexpression of BAFF receptors, as well as disturbed autocrine and paracrine BAFF network, seems to be related to inflammatory events and RA progression [1–6].

Although clinical development of BAFF antagonists as potential therapeutic target for systemic autoimmune conditions is promising, the benefit of specific agents such as belimumab, atacicept, or tabalumab in RA is controversial [2, 4, 6].

We systematically reviewed data from the literature focusing on the biology of BAFF, its homologue molecule APRIL and BAFF-binding receptors, dysregulation of BAFF/BAFF receptor signaling in RA and current status of targeting BAFF/BAFF receptor pathway.

2. BAFF and BAFF receptors physiology

2.1. BAF and APRIL

BAFF, also known as BLyS (B-lymphocyte stimulator), TALL-1 (TNF and apoptosis ligand-related leukocyte-expressed ligand 1), zTNF4, TNFSF13B (TNF ligand superfamily member 13B) or THANK, is a protein member of the TNF ligand family, critically involved in B-cell survival, maturation, and function [2–6]. As a vital cytokine for peripheral B-cell homeostasis, BAFF is acknowledged as a key regulator for both innate and adaptive immune responses [2–5].

Under normal conditions, BAFF is mainly expressed and secreted by a variety of cells including monocytes, dendritic cells, neutrophils, stromal cells, and activated T cells [2–14] and is typically upregulated by different cytokines, such as TNF-α, IFN-γ, and TGF-β [2–14].

BAFF is recognized under two isoforms, a biologically active full-length isoform and the alternatively spliced one, 4BAFF, meaning a protein with a small peptide deletion which does not bind to BAFF receptors, but has the ability to form heterotrimers with the original isoform [2–6]. Additionally, BAFF is expressed as a membrane-binding homotrimer and released as a soluble, biologically active molecule in peripheral blood after cleavage by a dedicated furinprotease [2, 4].

APRIL, a proliferation-inducing ligand known as the homolog molecule of BAFF or TNFSF13 (TNF ligand superfamily member 13), is also a key cytokine for B-cell activation and maturation; APRIL prompts B-cell proliferation, antibody class switching and survival, but is not required for the normal B-cell development [12–14].

Interestingly, BAFF and APRIL exhibit the ability to generate mixed molecules comprising BAFF/APRIL hetero-trimers [2–14] and TWE-PRIL (TNFSF12), an APRIL extracellular domain/TWEAK intracellular domain hybrid molecule [2, 4], as well as ΔBAFF, an alternatively spliced form of BAFF [4]. None of these molecules binds to BAFF receptors, but their co-expression with BAFF may have a deleterious impact on receptor signaling [2–14].

2.2. BAFF receptors signaling

Three distinct BAFF receptors typically expressed on B cells in different developmental stages are generally recognized: (i) BAFF receptor (BAFF-R, BR-3, TNFRSF13C or TNF receptor superfamily member 13C); (ii) transmembrane activator and calcium modulator ligand interactor (TACI, TNFRSF13B or TNF receptor superfamily member 13B); and (iii) B-cell maturation antigen (BCMA, TNFRSF17 or TNF receptor superfamily member 17) [2–14].

The expression of BAFF-binding receptors becomes evident only during the transitional stages of B-cells, varies according to the B-cell subset and is strictly dependent on various downstream mediators, further differentiation, maturation, and activation level as well [2–14]. Moreover, each receptor triggers its own set of signaling pathways [2, 4].

Thus, BAFF-R is essentially engaged in naïve and memory B-cell populations, with the highest expression in follicular and marginal zone B-lymphocytes, and is upregulated by B-cell receptor on mature B cells and enables most of the BAFF-dependent actions [2–14]. BAFF-R appears to be the most important receptor for mature B-cell survival and homeostasis in peripheral B cells [5].

TACI remains the predominant receptor on marginal zone B cells and short-lived plasma cells, while BCMA is typically expressed by long-lived plasma cells being essential for their optimal generation [2, 4]. The ability of TACI to act as a sink for BAFF, preventing the attachment of BAFF to its BAFF-R, may also reflect mixed regulatory functions on B cells [2, 4, 5, 10–14].

Although BAFF-R/BR3 stands as a specific receptor for both soluble and membrane-bound BAFF, TACI and BCMA can also bind to the homologous proliferation-inducing ligand APRIL [2, 4, 10–14].

Each of the three receptors has a different pattern of expression and mediates distinct functions [2, 4].

2.3. BAFF and BAFF receptors functioning

It is widely accepted that BAFF plays a crucial role in B-cell homeostasis, adjusting their maturation, proliferation, and survival under different backgrounds. BAFF may also indirectly interfere with T-cell functioning, providing several co-stimulatory signals in conjunction with T-cell receptor, mainly related to cellular proliferation and synthesis of mediators [2, 4].

Table 1 summarizes the BAFF/BAFF receptors functions in B and T cells (**Table 1**) [2–14].

Cell type	Function
B cells	Enhance B-cell and plasma cell survival Co-stimulate B-cell proliferation B-cell maturation Promote B-cell differentiation from transitional type 1 to type 2 cells Immunoglobulin synthesis T-cell-independent and T-cell-dependent antibody response
T cells	Enhance T-cell proliferation Enhance cytokine synthesis
Dendritic cells	Promote immune cell recruiting Promote cytokine synthesis

Source: Adapted from Ref. [2].

Table 1. Overview of main BAFF biological functions in immune cells.

2.3.1. BAFF and B-cell functioning

BAFF and APRIL mediate several important B-cell functions in normal settings, but dysregulated BAFF/BAFF receptors represent a significant event in different autoimmune conditions [2–14].

First, BAFF enhances long-term B-cell survival primarily through NF-kB pathway by upregulating anti-apoptotic Genes, particularly the expression of Bcl-2 gene family members [2–14]. While BAFF and APRIL typically improve the survival of plasmablasts, their role in promoting long-lived plasma cells persistence is still debatable [2, 4]. Moreover, either BAFF or APRIL accounts for the survival of plasma cells expressing TACI and/or BCMA [2, 4, 10–14]. By contrast, memory B cells do not require BAFF nor APRIL for their proliferation and survival [2, 4]. Thus, their survival and reactivation are both BAFF-independent [2, 4, 10–14]. Finally, BAFF-BAFF-R interface seems to be vital for the survival of B2 subpopulation from the transitional type 1 stage, with a minor input from TACI and without feedback from BCMA [2–14].

Second, BAFF enhances signaling through the B-cell receptor (BCR) by upregulating the expression of its co-receptors, namely CD21 and CD19, respectively [2–14]. The relation is bidirectional as BAFF-R expression is upregulated by B-cell receptor on mature B cells [2–14]. Additionally, there is a direct linkage between the intensity of BCR signaling and the extent of BAFF signal, particularly related to the non-classical NF-kB pathway which is operational for BAFF-R [2, 4–14]. Therefore, signaling through BAFF-R is able to promote B-lymphocytes survival in general, and individual late transitional and follicular B-cell survival [2–14].

Third, BAFF upregulates Toll-like receptor (TLR), endorses B-cell survival as well as Ig class switching and plasma cell differentiation [2–14]. The expression of BAFF-bound receptors on B cells, particularly TACI [2–14], is up-regulated via intracellular-activated TLR under the effect of specific immune complexes, with further relevance for augmented BCR-mediated signaling. Activated B cells by TLR-4 overexpress BAFF-R receptor types with subsequent susceptibility to apoptotic signals through Fas molecules [2–14].

Finally, the differentiation of peripheral autoreactive B cells depends on high BAFF levels [2–14].

2.3.2. BAFF and T-cell functioning: proliferation and cytokine production

While recent insights have extensively advanced our knowledge about BAFF/BAFF receptor intervention on B-cell activity in normal microenvironment and autoimmunity, the role of BAFF and APRIL in T-cell co-stimulation is still controversial [2, 4–14].

Classically, BAFF indirectly enhances T-cell proliferation [8] and arbitrates cytokine production, particularly during inflammation. Hence, the expansion of T-cell population may occur as a consequence of primary B-cell expansion/proliferation rather than a result of direct intervention of BAFF cytokine. Of interest, APRIL itself appears to mediate T-cell overflow [2–14]. T-cell-dependent immunoglobulin (Ig) responses strictly vary according to Ig subtype; IgM responses require BAFF intervention, whereas IgG responses are usually BAFF-independent [2–15]. Also, the intervention of BAFF receptors on T-cell function is debatable; while TACI might refashion T-cell functions, BAFF-R charge is unclear [2–14].

2.3.3. BAFF and dendritic cells functioning

It is increasingly recognized that BAFF influences dendritic cells to be actively involved in many physiologic as well as pathologic processes. Dendritic cells not only overexpress BAFF under different mediators (e.g., type I interferons) but also express BAFF receptors, predominantly TACI required for cellular proliferation and function [2–14]. The interaction between BAFF and dendritic cells stimulates immune cell trafficking and recruitment to inflammatory sites, and delivery of different cytokines and chemokines, mainly IL-1 and IL-6 [2–14].

3. BAFF and BAFF receptors in rheumatoid arthritis

Dysregulated BAFF/BAFF receptor signaling is clearly a trigger for autoimmunity in particular settings as is the case of systemic lupus erythematosus and RA [1, 2, 4, 5, 15–24]. To better understand the relevance of BAFF/BAFF receptor system in the complex pathobiology of RA with direct involvement in both early stages and disease progression, we emphasized several aspects regarding cell networking and BAFF influences, BAFF levels, and BAFF receptor expression in RA [2, 4, 15–24].

3.1. BAFF and BAFF receptor influences on cell networking in rheumatoid arthritis

We already mentioned the effects of BAFF in B- and T-cell biological homeostasis in general, and we further provide information on how BAFF and APRIL influence immune cells and resident synovial cells in RA [2, 4, 15–24].

RA is thought to be the result of an interplay between multiple cells and their products (cytokines and mediators), from both innate and adaptive immunity that lead to systemic inflammatory and tissue-damaging events [1–4].

Persistent immune cell trafficking into the inflamed joints typically focuses on B- and T-lymphocytes, with special polarization for TCD4+ subpopulation, neutrophils, macrophages, and dendritic cells, which actively infiltrate the RA synovium and orchestrate inflammation and cartilage damage [1–4]. At least three different histological subtypes of immune infiltrates are actually recognized within the RA synovitis, meaning diffuse, nodular infiltrates, and lymphoid aggregates with germinal centers [2–4].

Excess of pro-inflammatory cytokines (mainly TNF-α, IL-1β, IL-6, IL-15, IL-17, and IL-23) and other inflammatory mediators (prostaglandin E2, reactive oxygen Species, nitric oxide) together with tissue-degrading enzymes (matrix metalloproteinases and other enzymes synthetized by activated neutrophils) are essential performers, maintaining local cellular networking in RA joints [1–3].

As innate cytokines, BAFF and APRIL are potentially involved in the dysregulated immuno-inflammatory synovial microenvironment, affecting both autocrine and paracrine feedback [1–6]. In addition, BAFF and APRILL are involved in an amplification loop which is locally activated by inflammation: B- and T-lymphocytes, together with plasmacytoid and myeloid dendritic cells, are interconnected through a continuing crosstalk [1–4]. Thus, B cells migrated to the inflamed tissues and activated produce pro-inflammatory and destructive cytokines and chemokines, but also exert their potent effector function by presenting self-antigens to and activating T cells [2–4]. Moreover, immune complexes as a result of aberrant functioning of B cells induce the activation of different subtypes of dendritic cells within the IFN direct supervision and further enhance B- and T-participation [4].

3.1.1. Neutrophils, macrophages, dendritic cells, and B-lymphocyte loop in rheumatoid arthritis

It is clear that activated neutrophils, macrophages, as well as dendritic cells represent fundamental sources of BAFF in the inflamed RA joints; however, these cells may have variable importance in different RA stages, with neutrophils releasing BAFF in early RA, while macrophages in established disease [1–4, 14–24].

Abundant BAFF levels further support a positive feedback from B-lymphocytes, the BAFF/BAFF-R signaling being an important stimulator of B-cell proliferation, survival, and activation, with subsequent dysregulated B-cell functioning, with synthesis of various cytokines, and autoantibodies [1–4, 14–24].

Neutrophils incoming in the inflamed synovial joint is able to produce high levels of soluble BAFF under the direct action of TNF-α and local G-CSF [1–4]. Additionally, through BAFF-R reverse signaling [2–4], macrophages are able to enhance MMP-9 and other matrix-degrading mediators [2–4]. Dendritic cells express BAFF molecule in early RA stages and turn into mature dendritic cells, mediating B-cell proliferation [2–4] with subsequent increase in antigen presentation, antibody production, immune complex formation, and cytokine secretion [1–4].

3.1.2. Neutrophils, macrophages, dendritic cells, and T-lymphocytes loop in rheumatoid

BAFF may also interfere with T cells-dendritic cells interaction. BAFF is obviously involved in T helper 1 (Th1)-related immune responses [1–4, 14–24] and facilitates significant in situ CD4+ T-cell proliferation and Th1 as well as Th17 polarization [1–4]. Interestingly, pro-inflammatory cytokines such as IL-1, IL-6, and TNF-α are involved in upregulation of BAFF expression on various activated cells in the synovial microenvironment (macrophages, dendritic cells, neutrophils) enhancing Th17 polarization and subsequent synthesis of IL-17 cytokine [1–4].

3.1.3. Fibroblast-like macrophages, B- and T-cell loop in rheumatoid arthritis

Fibroblast-like macrophages are known to constitutively express BAFF in patients with RA, and BAFF expression is significantly upregulated under TNF-α and IFN-γ stimulation [2, 4]. Activated fibroblast-like macrophages are further able to secrete IL-6 and CXCL12, as well as adhesion molecules (VCAM-1) influencing the survival of mature B cells and synovial trafficking [2, 4]. Recent data suggest that CD4+ T cells under BAFF activation are able to induce the proliferation of fibroblast-like macrophages, with consequent overexpression of various pro-inflammatory cytokines, particularly TNF-α, IL-1β, and IL-6 [2–4, 14–24].

Overall, various residents as well as recruited cells in rheumatoid synovium are responsible for BAFF synthesis, especially dendritic cells, macrophages and fibroblast-like macrophages, neutrophils, and CD4+ T cells. Further, BAFF interventions on the effector cell network (dendritic cells, macrophages and fibroblast-like macrophages, neutrophils, TCD4+ lymphocytes, and B cells) are able to promote by positive feedback their differentiation, proliferation, activation with subsequent cytokine production, and survival [2, 4].

3.2. Abnormal BAFF levels in rheumatoid arthritis

Elevated levels of BAFF are found in several inflammatory diseases (lupus, Sjogren's, RA), and are related to disease activity [2–4]; RA exhibits a positive correlation between BAFF and disease activity, so that BAFF was recommended as a new index of RA activity [2, 4, 14–24].

Interestingly, a recent study designates BAFF as a predictor of RA prognosis and outcomes as serum level of BAFF parallels radiographic progression and higher plasma BAFF correlates with advanced radiographic joint damage [2, 4, 14–24].

Elevated levels of both BAFF and APRIL along with their receptors in patients with RA, particularly in rheumatoid factor (RF) positive, anti-cyclic citrullinated peptide antibodies (ACPA)-positive subtype, active, erosive disease, support their role in the pathobiology of the disease [2, 4, 14–24]. Although abnormal BAFF was typically found in both serum and synovial fluid in RA, significantly higher synovial levels suggest local BAFF production, driving the maturation as well as preserving autoreactive B cells within the inflamed tissue, with subsequent amplification of inflammatory processes and generation of autoantibodies [2, 4, 14–24]. Furthermore, seropositive RA status is clearly associated with higher concentrations of BAFF than seronegative disease [2–4, 14–24], and there is a statistically significant correlation Between RF titer and BAFF level [2–4, 14–24].

Finally, it seems that BAFF levels depend on RA stage, and disease duration as well [2, 4, 14–24]; thereby, patients with very early RA (disease duration less than 6 weeks) have highest BAFF levels, followed by those with established (lasting more than 12 months) and long-standing disease [2, 4, 14–24]. Undifferentiated early arthritis also has lower BAFF levels as compared to very early RA supporting a role for BAFF in the initial steps of disease development [2, 4, 14–24].

However, local BAFF overexpression in RA joints is independent of the histologic subtype of RA synovitis (diffuse, nodular, and germinal center) [2, 4, 14–24]. BAFF also contributes to local B-lymphocyte function and survival, their activation and differentiation with subsequent production of autoantibodies [2, 4, 14–24]. Moreover, BAFF induces an autoreactive B-cell polarization as stressed by several studies in experimental arthritis models [2, 4, 14–24]. Thus, there is an interrelation between BAFF levels and humoral immune response [2, 4, 14–24], particularly RF, ACPA, as well as circulating immune complexes [2, 4, 14–24].

3.3. Abnormal expression of BAFF receptors in rheumatoid arthritis

BAFF receptors are also altered in RA [2, 4, 14–24]. The three receptor subtypes are expressed as follows: TACI-excessive levels are detected during first steps of RA development (early RA), BAFF-R has an obvious increase with disease progression, while BCMA expression has the same pattern as healthy population [2, 4, 14–24]. Furthermore, TACI receptor distribution and expression are typically lower than BAFF-R/BR3, without any relation with the histological subtype of synovitis [2, 4, 14–24]. On the other hand, it seems that only BCMA and its gene expression correlate with different patterns of B- and T-cell distribution among the synovial tissue [2, 4, 14–24]. Thereby, BCMA is significantly enhanced in synovial tissue presenting with follicular lymphocyte aggregation with or without germinal centers formation than in diffuse lymphoid infiltration synovitis [2, 4, 14–24]. Finally, aberrant expression of BCMA in resident synovial cells, Fibroblast-like synoviocytes, was reported in RA [2, 4, 14–24].

4. Targeting BAFF and BAFF receptors for rheumatoid arthritis

Accumulating data on the importance of B cells in various autoimmune diseases have reshaped the therapeutic armamentarium, specifically directed toward B-lymphocytes [2, 4, 25, 26].

While playing a pivotal role in B-cell survival and functioning, BAFF/BAFF receptor system recently emerged as a reasonable target for different autoimmune conditions [2, 4, 25, 26]; furthermore, several BAFF antagonists are already under development exploring the appropriate therapeutic intervention based on BAFF blockade in RA [2, 4, 25, 26].

Generally, therapeutic BAFF antagonism accounts not only for direct B-cell depletion and indirect impairment of B-cell-mediated processes such as antigen presentation, cytokine synthesis, and humoral immune response, but may also influence T-cell biology based on co-stimulatory signals [2, 4, 25, 26].

http://dx.doi.org/10.5772/66580

Several mechanisms were proposed to explain potential efficacy of BAFF/BAFF receptors antagonists in autoimmune conditions [2, 4, 25, 26]: (i) substantial B-cell depletion, particularly for bone-marrow-derived B2 subpopulation, known to undergo BAFF-mediated differentiation into follicular cells or marginal zone B cells [2, 4, 25, 26]; (ii) impaired immunoglobulin synthesis, especially in newly emerging B cells, while established memory B cells are spared; decreased transitional B-cell survival along with disturbed B-cell receptor co-signaling may further support altered immunoglobulin repertoire [2, 4, 25, 26]; (iii) indirect effect on other cells belonging to the BAFF amplification loop (T cells, dendritic cells, and macrophages) and their inflammatory mediators promoting decreased antigen presentation, decreased epitope spreading, immune complexes formation, and cytokine synthesis [2, 4, 25, 26]; (iv) selective depletion of plasmablasts expressing different BAFF-binding receptors [2, 4, 25, 26].

At least two classes of BAFF antagonists are currently recognized including (i) BAFF-blockers or monoclonal anti-BAFF antibodies (e.g., belimumab and tabalumab) and (ii) receptor fusion proteins (e.g., atacicept), specifically binding soluble BAFF, membrane BAFF, or APRIL [2, 4, 25, 26].

A simplified view of BAFF/APRIL/BAFF-binding receptor pathway and their targeted therapy in immune mediated is presented (**Figure 1**).

We reviewed the current status of targeting BAFF/BLyS, APRIL and their receptors in RA.

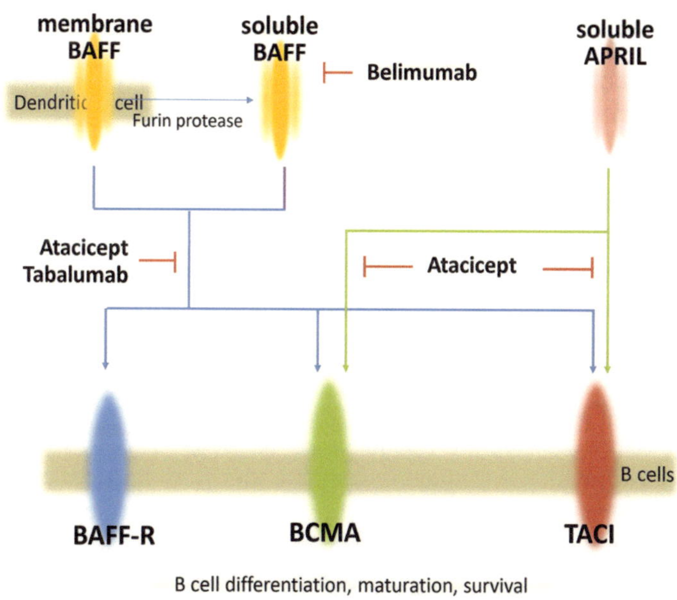

Figure 1. BAFF/APRIL/BAFF-binding receptor pathway and targeted therapy. Source: Adapted from Vincent F. et al., Nat Rev Rheum. 2014; Ref. [43].

4.1. Belimumab

Belimumab, the first targeted biological therapy for systemic lupus erythematosus, is a recombinant fully human immunoglobulin G subclass 1 (IgG1k) anti-BAFF monoclonal antibody recently approved for antinuclear antibody-positive lupus, selectively targeting soluble BAFF, but not membrane-bound BAFF or other members of the TNF ligand family. Moreover, belimumab demonstrates inhibitory activity on all three BAFF receptors (TACI, BCMA, BR3) with equivalent potency [2, 4, 26–30].

BAFF overexpression in RA theoretically induces local (synovial) autoreactive B-cell proliferation and survival. Preventing BAFF from binding to B cells is able to impair B-cell-mediated autoimmune response and could be an attractive target for RA patients [2, 4, 26–30].

The efficacy and tolerability of a novel, fully human variant of anti-BLyS monoclonal antibody was further evaluated in patients with active RA non-responsive to standard therapy in different clinical trials [2, 4, 26–30]. While safety data are convincing across all the studies and belimumab seems to be a promising agent for a specific RA population, optimal clinical efficacy needs further evaluation [2, 4, 26–30]. The majority of trials have demonstrated positive outcomes under belimumab BAFF-blockade, meaning significant response rates according to American College of Rheumatology (ACR) improvement ≥20% criteria but not ACR50 or ACR70, specifically for RA patients classified as having high disease activity (disease activity score DAS28>5.1), RF and ACPA-positive status, naïve to other biologics including TNF antagonists, previous methotrexate failure or low baseline BAFF levels [2, 4, 26–30].

4.2. Tabalumab

Tabalumab, formerly LY2127399, is another fully human IgG4 anti-BAFF monoclonal antibody that binds to and neutralizes soluble and membrane-bound BAFF, but not to APRIL [2, 4, 25, 31–35].

Efficacy and safety of tabalumab in active RA despite ongoing methotrexate was assessed in several phase 2 and 3 randomized-controlled studies and their open-label extensions performed on diverse patient populations comprising either bio-naive or bio-experienced RA with an inadequate response to TNF inhibitors (non-responders or intolerant) [2, 4, 25, 31–35]. Clinical efficacy parameters included standardized measures such as ACR20, ACR50, and ACR70 improvement criteria, DAS28-C-reactive protein (DAS28-CRP), and Health Assessment Questionnaire-Disability Index (HAQ-DI), while total B-cell counts or CD3-CD20 B cells and serum immunoglobulins were used for biological impact [2, 4, 25, 31–35]. Of interest, each one of the four phase 2 clinical trials (identifier NCT00308282, NCT00689728, NCT00785928, and NCT00837811) provided encouraging results under flexible doses of anti-BAFF and a background of stable methotrexate, with meaningful clinical and biological RA improvement as compared to placebo, regardless of prior treatment [2, 4, 25, 31–35]. However, tabalumab received no further validation following two phase 3 randomized, double-blind, placebo-controlled studies aiming to demonstrate drug efficacy and safety in patients with moderate-to-severe RA with inadequate response to one or more TNF inhibitors [25, 30, 34–36]. The interim analyses prompted the withdrawal of tabalumab due to lack of efficacy, not to safety concerns [2, 4, 25, 31–35].

To summarize, although tabalumab showed clinical and biological efficacy in phase 2 clinical trials irrespective of prior exposure to synthetic remissive drugs (methotrexate) or biologics, phase 3 trials fail to promote clinical benefit in patients with moderate-to-severe RA with prior inadequate response to TNF antagonists. Despite demonstrating biological improvement as supported by substantial change in B-cell count and decline in serum immunoglobulin levels, it is obvious that targeting the BAFF pathway alone is not a feasible strategy in RA [2, 4, 25, 31–35].

4.3. Atacicept

Atacicept is a recombinant fusion protein between the extracellular domain of one of the BAFF receptors (TACI) and the Fc portion of human IgG1, able to inhibit B-cell maturation, differentiation, and survival, as well as immunoglobulin synthesis by disconnecting B cells from standardized growth and development signals [2, 4, 25, 36–41]. In contrast to BAFF monoclonal antibodies, atacicept not only binds to and neutralizes BAFF but also targets APRIL molecule [2, 4, 25, 36–41] and could be an efficient target for RA treatment by inhibiting activation of TACI-mediated signaling [2, 4, 25, 36–42].

Preclinical and phase 1 clinical studies showed promising results as atacicept was well tolerated, with no increased incidence of infections, and displayed a meaningful biological activity with impaired levels of immunoglobulin, RF and ACPA, and a biphasic response in B-cell count [2, 4, 25, 36–41]. Moreover, atacicept induced substantial clinical improvement, despite the nonlinear pharmacokinetic profile [2, 4, 25, 36–41].

Nevertheless, AUGUST I (Clinical Trials.gov: NCT00430495) and AUGUST II (Clinical Trials.gov: NCT00595413), two phase 2 clinical trials, failed to demonstrate the efficacy of atacicept in moderate-to-severe RA patients. Both studies were specifically designed to assess efficacy, safety, and biological activity of atacicept in RA with an inadequate response to TNF inhibitors (AUGUST I) [2, 4, 25, 36–41] or biologically naive patients suboptimally controlled or intolerant to classic remissive agents (methotrexate) [2, 4, 25, 36–41].

Although the primary efficacy end point (ACR20 response) was not achieved in none of phase 2 studies, atacicept significantly reduced the immunoglobulin (IgM, IgG, and IgA) and rheumatoid factor levels in a dose-dependent manner. The safety profile was acceptable as atacicept did not show an increased susceptibility to infections, although the overall rate of adverse events was somewhat higher than placebo and lupus [2, 4, 25, 36–41].

To summarize, despite clinical and biological efficacy expressed in preclinical arthritis models and phase 1 clinical trial, phase 2 studies with atacicept fail to promote clinical benefit in patients with moderate-to-severe RA with inadequate response to either prior TNF antagonists or methotrexate [2, 4, 25, 36–41].

4.4. Other BAFF antagonists (AMG-623 and BR3-Fc)

Other BAFF-blockade agents are under development, targeting different BAFF receptor-binding molecules. A good example is A-623, previously known as AMG-623, a polypeptide fusion protein containing both IgG and the ligand-binding section of the BAFF-R, able to block both membrane and soluble BAFF and, therefore, to impair normal B-cell functioning

[43]. Briobacept or BR3-Fc is another distinct BAFF-blocking molecule acting as a homodimeric fusion glycoprotein including the extracellular ligand-binding portion of BAFF-R and the Fc portion of an IgG. This new drug was typically designed to induce further B-cell apoptosis interfering with BAFF/BAFF-R signaling [2, 4, 43].

5. Conclusions

Abnormal BAFF signaling (throughout either overexpression of B-cell-related activation and survival genes, or BAFF receptors) represents an important step in the pathobiology of rheumatoid arthritis, particularly by promoting the development of autoreactive B cells in early disease, but also by supporting disease progression.

Although BAFF/APRIL/BAFF receptors targeting therapy seems to be an attractive option for systemic autoimmune conditions, particularly systemic lupus erythematosus, considerable response heterogeneity and safety concerns are reported in rheumatoid arthritis.

Author details

Codrina Ancuta[1]*, Cristina Pomirleanu[1], Claudia Mihailov[2], Eugen Ancuta[3] and Daniela Opris[4]

*Address all correspondence to: codrina_ancuta@yahoo.com

1 Rheumatology Department, Clinical Rehabilitation Hospital, Rheumatology 2 Department, 'Grigore T. Popa' University of Medicine and Pharmacy, Iasi, Romania

2 Clinical Port Hospital of Constanta, Faculty of Medicine, 'Ovidius' University of Constanta, Constanta, Romania

3 'Elena Doamna' Cinical Hospital, Research Department, Iasi, Romania

4 Internal Medicine and Rheumatology Department, 'Sfanta Maria' University Hospital, 'Carol Davila' University of Medicine and Pharmacy, Bucuresti, Romania

References

[1] Bugatti S, Vitolo B, Caporali R, et al. Cells in rheumatoid arthritis: from pathogenic players to disease biomarkers. BioMed Res Int. 2014;**2014**:681678 (1–14).

[2] Wei F, Chang Y, Wei W. The role of BAFF in the progression of rheumatoid arthritis. Cytokine. 2015;**76**(2):537–544.

[3] Moura RA, Graca L, Fonseca JE. To B or not to B conductor of rheumatoid arthritis orchestra. Clinic Rev Allerg Immunol. 2012;**43**(3):281–291.

[4] Ramanujam M, Davidson A. The current status of targeting BAFF/BLyS for autoimmune. Arthritis Res Ther. 2004;**6**:197–202.

[5] Woo YJ, Yoon BY, Jhun JY, et al. Regulation of B cell activating factor (BAFF) receptor expression by NF-κB signaling arthritis B cells. Exp Mol Med. 2011;**43**(6):350–357.

[6] Striz I, Brabcova E, Kolesar L, et al. Cytokine networking of innate immunity cells: a potential target of therapy. Clin Sci. 2014;**126**(9):593–612.

[7] Davidson A. Targeting BAFF in autoimmunity. Curr Opin Immunol. 2010;**22**:732–739.

[8] Lin Z, Davidson A. BAFF and selection of autoreactive B cells. Trends Immunol. 2011;**32**(8):388–394.

[9] Pillai S, Mattoo H, Cariappa A. B cells and autoimmunity. Curr Opin Immunol. 2011;**23**(6):721–731.

[10] Liu Z, Davidson A. BAFF inhibition: a new class of drugs for the treatment of autoimmunity. Exp Cell Res. 2011;**317**(9):1270–1277.

[11] Mackay F, Schneider P, Rennert P, et al. BAFF and APRIL: a tutorial on B cell. Ann Rev Immunol. 2003;**21**:231–264.

[12] Martin F, Kearney JF. B-cell subsets and the mature preimmune repertoire. Marginal zone and B1 B cells as part of a 'natural immune memory'. Immunol Rev. 2000;**175**:70–79.

[13] Marckay F, Mackay CR. The role of BAFF in B-cell maturation. T-cell activation and autoimmunity. Trends Immunol. 2002;**23**(3):1113–1125.

[14] Moisini L, Davidson A. BAFF: a local and systemic target in autoimmune diseases. Clin Exp Immunol. 2009;**1582**(2):155–163.

[15] De la Torre I, Moura RA, Leandro MJ, et al. B-cell-activating factor expression on naïve and memory B cells: relationship with relapse in patients with rheumatoid arthritis following B-cell depletion therapy. Ann Rheum Dis. 2010;**69**:2181–2188.

[16] Dong W, Li X, Liu Zhu P. Infiltrations of plasma cells in synovium are highly associated with synovial fluid levels of APRIL in inflamed peripheral joints of rheumatoid arthritis. Rheumatol Int. 2009;**29**:801–806.

[17] Geng Y, Zhang ZL. Comparative study on the level of B lymphocyte stimulator (BlyS) and frequency of lymphocytes between sero-negative and sero-positive rheumatoid arthritis patients. Int J Rheuma. 2012;**15**(5):478–485.

[18] Tan SM, Xu D, Roschke V, et al. Local production of B lymphocyte stimulator protein and APRIL in arthritic joints of patients with inflammatory arthritis. Arthritis Rheum. 2003;**48**(4):982–992.

[19] Seyler TM, Park YW, Takemura S, et al. BLyS and APRIL in rheumatoid arthritis. J Clin Invest. 2005;**115**(11):3083–3092.

[20] Nakajima K, Itoh K, Nagatani K, et al. Expression of BAFF and BAFF-R in the synovial tissue of patients with rheumatoid arthritis. Scand J Rheumatol. 2007;**36**:365–372.

[21] Leandro MJ, Cambridge G. Expression of B cell activating factor (BAFF) and BAFF-binding receptors in rheumatoid arthritis. J Rheumatol. 2013;**8**:1247–1250.

[22] Moura RA, Canhão H, Polido-Pereira J, et al. BAFF and TACI gene expression are increased in patients with untreated very early rheumatoid arthritis. J Rheumatol. 2013;**40**(8):1293–1302.

[23] Moura RA, Cascão R, Perpétuo I, et al. Cytokine pattern in very early rheumatoid arthritis favours B-cell activation and survival. Rheumatology. 2011;**50**(2):278–282.

[24] Moura RA, Weinmann P, Pereira PA, et al. Alternations on peripheral blood B-cell subpopulations in very early arthritis. Rheumatology. 2010;**49**:1082–1092.

[25] Blüml S, McKeever K, Ettinger R, et al. B-cell targeted therapeutics in clinical development. Arthritis Res Ther. 2013;15(1):54.

[26] Stohl W, Scholz JL, Cancro MP. Targeting BLyS in rheumatic disease: the sometimes – bumpy road from bench to bedside. Curr Opin Rheumatol. 2011;23(305-310)

[27] Jin X, Ding C. Belimumab –an anti-BLyS human monoclonal antibody for Rheumatoid Arthritis. Expert Opin Biol Ther. 2013;13(2):315-322.

[28] Eli Lilly and Company. ttps://newsroom.lilly.com/releasedetail.cfm?ReleaseID=738769. Press Release 2013 [Internet]. 2013 [Updated: 2013]. [Accessed: 26.08.2016]

[29] Genovese M, Filipowicz-Sosnowska A, Merrill J, et al. Differential responsiveness to belimumab in combination with standard of care therapy in RF+, TNF-inhibitors and methotrexate partial responder of subjects with moderate-severe rheumatoid arthritis. Arthritis Rheum. 2005;52:s1989.

[30] Stohl W, Merrill JT, McKay JD, et al. Efficacy and safety of belimumab in patients with rheumatoid arthritis: a phase II, randomized, double-blind, placebo-controlled, dose-ranging Study. J Rheumatol. 2013;40(5):579-589.

[31] Combe B, van Vollenhoven. Novel targeted therapies: the future of rheumatoid arthritis? Mavrilumab and tabalumab as examples. Ann Rheum Dis. 2013; 72 (9):1433-1435.

[32] Genovese MC, Fleischmann RM, Greenwald M, et al . Tabalumab, an anti-BAFF monoclonal antibody, in patients with active rheumatoid arthritis with an inadequate response to TNF inhibitors. Ann Rheum Diss. 2013;72(9):1461-1468.

[33] Greenwald M, Szczepanski L, Kennedy A, et al. A 52-week, open-label study evaluating the safety and efficacy of tabalumab, an anti-B-cell activating factor monoclonal antibody, for rheumatoid arthritis. Arthritis Res Ther. 2014;**16**(4):415–425.

[34] Smolen JS, Weinblatt ME, van der Heijde D, et al. Efficacy and safety of tabalumab, an anti-B-cell-activating factor monoclonal antibody, in patients with rheumatoid arthritis who had an inadequate response to methotrexate therapy: results from a phase III multicenter, randomized, double-blind study. Ann Rheum Dis. 2015; 74:1567-1570.

[35] Genovese MC, Lee E, Satterwhite J, et al. A phase 2 dose-ranging study of subcutaneous tabalumab for the treatment of patients with active rheumatoid arthritis and an inadequate response to methotrexate. Ann Rheum Dis. 2013;**72**(9):1453–1460.

[36] Genovese MC, Kinnaman N, de La Bourdonnave G, et al. Atacicept in patients with rheumatoid arthritis and an inadequate response to tumor necrosis factor antagonist therapy: results of a phase II, randomized, placebo-controlled, dose- finding trial. Arthritis Rheum. 2011;**63**(7):1793–1803.

[37] Nanda S. Therapy: Atacicept lacks clinical efficacy in RA. Nat Rev Rheumatol. 2011;**7**(6):313.

[38] Richez C, Truchetet ME, Schaeverbeke T, et al. Atacicept as an investigated therapy for rheumatoid arthritis. Expert Opin Investig. 2014;**23**(9):1285–1294.

[39] Bracewell C, Isaacs JD, Emery P, et al. Atacicept, a novel B cell-targeting biological therapy for the treatment of rheumatoid arthritis. Expert Opin Biol Ther. 2009;**9**(7):909–919.

[40] Tak PP, Thurlings RM, Rossier C, et al. Atacicept on patients with rheumatoid arthritis: results of a multicenter, phase Ib, double-blind, placebo-controlled, dose-escalating, single- and repeated-dose study. Arthritis Rheum. 2008;**58**:61–72.

[41] Van Vollenhoven RF, Kinnman N, Vincent E, et al. Atacicept in patients with rheumatoid arthritis and an inadequate response to methotrexate: results of a phase II, randomized, placebo- controlled trial. Arthritis Rheum. 2011;**63**(7):1782–1792.

[42] Hsu H, Khare SD, Lee F, et al. A novel modality of BAFF-specific inhibitor AMG623 peptibody reduces B-cell number and improves outcomes in murine models of autoimmune disease. Clin Exp Rheumatol. 2012;**30**(2):197–201.

[43] Nakayamada S, Tanaka Y. BAFF- and APRIL-targeted therapy in systemic autoimmune diseases. Inflamm Regener. 2016;36:6.

Section 3

Microbes and Rheumatoid Arthritis

Chapter 5

The Gut Microbiota and Inflammation in Rheumatoid Arthritis

Reem Hamdy A. Mohammed and
Hesham Ibrahim I. Elmakhzangy

Additional information is available at the end of the chapter

http://dx.doi.org/10.5772/67368

Abstract

"Mutualism" is a well-defined relationship that describes a form of cooperation between two living organisms of different species that ends up with a beneficial outcome for each one. Any disruption to such a relationship by an external trigger or a potential intruder puts at risk the well-being of both. In humans, oral and gut microbiota provide a noteworthy model of beneficial mutualism. Multiple recent evidences point to the possible pathologic consequences of a disruption to this ecosystem (altered microbiota profile or dysbiosis) on human well-being. The gut-joint axis found its clear way "Proof of Principle" in the pathogenesis of autoimmune rheumatic diseases including rheumatoid arthritis (RA), seronegative spondyloarthropathies, and Behcet's disease in a number of studies. Current therapeutic trends are directed towards the diverse biologic and immune-pathogenic factors involved in the disease process. Addressing dysbiosis in RA features an attractive future therapeutic target. In this chapter, authors aim to explore the recent evidences regarding the pathogenic role of "gut dysbiosis" in rheumatoid arthritis (RA), highlighting the spectrum of immune-pathogenic events that might contribute to disease evolution and inspecting future directives of research.

Keywords: Mutualism, microbiota, dysbiosis, pathogenesis, autoimmune rheumatic diseases, rheumatoid arthritis

1. Rheumatoid Arthritis and The Microbiome Theory "The Revival of an Old Hypothesis"

Rheumatoid arthritis (RA) is a systemic immune-mediated chronic inflammatory disease that predominantly targets diarthrodial joints contributing to synovial inflammation, joint destruction, and deformity. The disease has been initially recognized as a complex genetically based inflammatory joint disease, a concept that was redefined toward a multifactorial immune-mediated etiology. The etiopathogenesis of rheumatoid arthritis is typically a challenge incorporating complex network of genetic factors (HLA genes), environmental and biological factors (infections, a dominant pro-inflammatory profile, dysbiosis), as well as individual habits (smoking) interacting to shape up disease phenotype [1, 2].

An infectious etiology of RA has been proposed for decades, Banntyne and Wohlmann in 1896 were the first to suggest a mycobacterial etiology behind the development of rheumatoid arthritis, a theory that awaited solid scientific evidence. The hypothesis of "molecular mimicry" and cross-reactivity between epitopes of microbial origin with a self-protein was among the proposed mechanisms to explain the role of infectious agents in the breakdown of immune tolerance in RA. Certain viral infections like Epstein-Barr virus (EBV), cytomegalovirus (CMV), and Parvovirus B19 have been additionally claimed as potential etiopathogenic agents in RA [3–9].

1.1. The oral sepsis hypothesis

In the 1900s, the oral sepsis hypothesis and its relation to arthritis led to the use of teeth extraction as a prevalent treatment of disease for several decades. The impact of polymicrobial phylotypes and the pro-inflammatory burden in periodontitis proved its contribution to the pro-inflammatory drive in RA. The *Porphyromonas gingivalis*, a Gram-negative anaerobe bacterium and part of periodontopathic microbiome, contributes to protein citrullination, which leads to anticitrullinated autoantibody (ACPA) formation and joint inflammation in RA [6–13].

The infectious profile further extended to include other pathogenic bacterial species as wells as cell membrane proteins of mycoplasma in RA like *Proteus mirabilis* (*sharing sequence similarities to peptide sequences at amino acid position 67–74 of the HLA-shared epitope in RA and bacterial-specific antibodies detected in sera of RA patients*) [14, 15]. The presence of specific *Escherichia coli*, *Mycoplasma fermentans*, and *Klebsiella pneumonia* in the gut has been associated with RF positivity and has been linked to inflammatory arthritis in many ethnic populations [16].

1.2. The infectious hypothesis and therapeutic evidences

The relationship between infections and arthritis was indirectly reinforced by the time antimicrobials showed an observable beneficial effect in the amelioration of arthritis. In the 1940s, sulfasalazine was the first rationally designed drug in the field of rheumatology, where RA was thought to be caused by Streptococci found in milk. Sulfasalazine was designed as a deliberate attempt to combine a sulfonamide antibiotic with a salicylate anti-inflammatory agent through an azo bond. Such "combination therapy" brought up good initial responses in RA as well as enteropathies. The triple DMARD therapy (a combination of methotrexate, sulfasalazine and hydroxychloroquine) currently stands among the first few recommendations in RA patients with poor prognostic features and moderate to high levels of disease activity [17–21].

http://dx.doi.org/10.5772/67368

Certain antibiotics like tetracycline have proven efficacy in the treatment of early seropositive RA which led to the approval of minocycline, as a DMARD [22, 23]. Clarithromycin is another example that gave observable beneficial effects in some refractory cases [24]. Treatment with probiotics, particularly *Bifidobacterium, Lactobacillus,* and *Faecalibacterium prausnitzii,* showed protective effects in NSAID-treated animal models of arthritis. Theories regarding supplementations of microbiome-derived molecules with immune-modulating properties (e.g., Polysaccharide A, short-chain fatty acids) provide promising novel immune regulatory effects by possibly downregulating pro-inflammatory cytokines with upregulation of the anti-inflammatory profile [25–27].

2. The human gut ecosystem

Mutualism is a well-defined relationship between living organisms. The term describes a form of cooperation between two living organisms of different species that ends up with a beneficial outcome for each one. Partners in a mutualistic relationship make headway together with each forming a part of the other's environment and maintaining its homeostasis in a typically harmless yet useful way. A disruption to such a relationship by an external trigger or a potential intruder puts at risk the well-being of both. In humans, oral and gut microbiota provide a noteworthy model of beneficial mutualism. Multiple recent evidences point to the possible pathologic consequences of a disruption to this ecosystem (altered microbiota profile or dysbiosis) on human well-being. The gut-joint axis found its clear way "Proof of Principle" in the pathogenesis of autoimmune rheumatic diseases including RA, seronegative spondyloarthropathies, and Behcet's disease in a number of studies.

The term "microbiota" is defined as the ecological community of symbiotic, commensal, and pathogenic microorganisms that literally inhabit the human body and effectively contribute to human health and might contribute to disease. According to their contributions to human health, they can be classified to symbiomes and pathobiomes. The symbiome microbiota are groups of microorganisms predominantly bacterial as well as fungal (previously recognized as normal flora) that get acquired at birth and inhabit every part of the human body from the skin to mucosa (mouth, eyes, gut, and genital tracts). The alimentary tract represents an established microbial habitat for almost 29–30% of the overall commensal/symbiome population in the human body. They involve over 500 bacterial species encoding around three million different genes constituting a complex challenging ecosystem, difficult to differentially analyze or understand [28, 29].

2.1. The development of the human microbiota profile

The general composition of gut microbiota is much similar in most healthy individuals; however, the individuals' microbiota profile retains a highly personalized pattern (fingerprint). This pattern helps to keep in situ homeostasis in healthy individuals; therefore triggers of dysbiosis are expected to offer a threat to the humans' well-being in a variety of forms.

At birth: The initial shape up of the different microbial colonies of the gut begins as early as childbirth by the time the newborn gets exposed to microorganisms that inhabit the maternal genital tract during normal vaginal delivery (first encounter), maternal fecal bacteria, or the skin in the case of caesarian section. The fetal fingerprint of microbiota gets additionally shaped up by the skin as well as breast milk microbiota that add their signature to this microbial network [30].

Adulthood: The typical adult microbiota profile emerges by the end of the first year with more than 1000 different species from a dozen different divisions colonizing the gastrointestinal tract (4×10^{13} colonizing bacteria). The profile becomes increasingly stable with age. The acquired bacterial species pass through a series of modifications with colonies competing for survival, alternating their dominance aiming to establish phylogenetic richness and species diversity at the same time. Serial microbial evolutions are proven to be largely dependent on a multiplicity of host as well as environmental factors (the host genetics, the maternal microbiota, and mode of delivery as major determinants). Breast milk composition is another proven shaping factor of individuals' microbiota profile (*Bifidobacterium* is among the dominant gut microbiota in breast-fed infants compared to artificially fed ones and is deficient in patients with RA). Aging; lifestyle patterns including diet, smoking, and obesity; and infections also contribute [31–34].

2.2. The identification and characterization of gut microbiota

The human microbiome project served as a major contributor toward better understanding of the human microbiome. For a sufficient period of time, the conventional culture-based methods were the only methods available and routinely used for identification of gut microbiota, with over 500 bacterial species successfully isolated, cultured, and characterized from the human GI tract [35].

The majority of gut microbiota (over 80%) could not be technically cultivated ranking the culture-based methods as an investigative technique of limited value in determining the actual microbial diversity. The revolutionary era of the human microbiome project announced in 2007 and the utilization of novel culture-independent molecular techniques have successfully contributed to the in-depth understanding of such complex human microbiome network. Such culture-independent techniques target the highly conserved 16S ribosomal RNA (rRNA) gene sequence (a component the 30S subunit of prokaryotic ribosomes) of bacterial and archaeal microorganisms. Universal PCR primers targeting these conserved regions can be used for gene amplification to provide the complete nucleotide sequence of the 16S rRNA without prior knowledge of which bacterial species are present. Concomitantly, the 16S rRNA gene also contains hypervariable regions that provide species-specific signature sequences and enable unbiased bacterial identification utilizing next-generation sequencing platforms. Examples of these molecular techniques include quantitative polymerase chain reaction (qPCR), temperature or denaturing gradient gel electrophoresis (TGGE or DGGE), terminal-restriction fragment length polymorphism (T-RFLP), and fluorescent in situ hybridization (FISH). The next-generation sequencing and phylogenetic microarrays promote the in-depth analysis of the complete phylogenetic diversity of the intestinal microbiota, whereas the whole-genome shotgun sequencing is a technique currently applied for identification of the metabolic and enzymatic pathways present in these microbial communities. Such techniques were able to identify a portion of predominant species in the human gut [36–38].

http://dx.doi.org/10.5772/67368

Genomic culture-independent techniques disclosed that the human intestine is dominated by two divisions of bacteria, Bacteroidetes and Firmicutes, and both contribute to more than two-thirds of the total gut microbiota including anaerobes such as *Bacteroides*, *Porphyromonas*, *Bifidobacterium*, *Lactobacillus*, and *Clostridium* [13, 34, 39, 40].

2.3. The human-microbiota interdependence

Microbiota are involved in a number of structural, biological, protective, and metabolic processes including angiogenesis, postnatal intestinal maturation, and xenobiotic metabolism. They are additionally involved in the synthesis of vitamins, the digestion, and uptake of nutrients. Microbiota are capable of metabolically simplifying nutritional components through the process of fermentation; an important example is the indigestible carbohydrates (complex starch and dietary fibers) as well as short-chain fatty acids (SCFA, e.g., acetate, butyrate, and propionate) which constitute a critical prerequisite in a number of host physiological functions [41].

2.3.1. Microbiota and immunity

A unique harmonious and complex interplay exists between gut microbiota and the local as well as the systemic immune response in humans. Colonizing microbiota and their products have a profound effect on the development and maintenance of the immune system integrity [42–45].

2.3.1.1. The microbiota and T-cell differentiation, proliferation, and functions

Evidences support the existence of immune cross talks between the microbiota-derived products and the gut epithelium that involves molecular exchange of bacterial signals recognized by host receptors to mediate beneficial outcomes for both the microbiome and human beings [42–47]. The gut microbiota have the potential to effectively stimulate and direct the host innate and adaptive immune responses in humans by triggering instructional signals to the immune cells, particularly regulatory T (Treg)-cell and T-helper (Th) cell differentiation.

2.3.1.2. Short-chain fatty acids and Treg cells

SCFAs are actively produced by anaerobic microbiota in the colon as fermentation products of digestion-resistant dietary fibers [46, 47]. SCFAs produced locally in the colon are either absorbed and metabolized within the colonocytes or transported into the circulation to reach other organs, such as the liver and muscles. SCFAs exert direct and indirect regulatory effects on epithelial cells, antigen-presenting cells, and T cells via multiple mechanisms including metabolic regulation, histone deacetylase inhibition (HDAC inhibition), and G-protein–coupled receptor (GPCR) activation.

SCFAs can be converted to Acetyl-CoA and integrated into the citric acid cycle (Krebs cycle). Acetyl-CoA is a central molecule that stores energy and is eventually oxidized to CO_2 for energy production (the cellular energy [ATP/ADP] level increases). This boosts a homeostatic T-cell sensor mammalian target of rapamycin (mTOR) to be activated in T cells which skews T-cell differentiation into effector T cells such as Th1 and Th17 cells at the expense of $FoxP3^+$ T cells. mTOR activation also promotes the generation of $IL\text{-}10^+$ cells. Thus, the SCFA regulation of cell metabolism and mTOR accounts for the increased generation of Th1 cells, Th17 cells, and IL-10$^+$ cells.

The activation of SCFA-binding G-protein–coupled receptors (GPCRs) such as GPR41, GPR43, GPR109A, and Olfr78 initiates T-cell differentiation.

All major SCFAs such as C2, C3, C4, and C5 have HDAC inhibitor activity. Class I/II HDACs are major targets of SCFA inhibition in a concentration-dependent pattern. Treg generation was increased as a result of HDAC inhibition by SCFAs and histone H3 acetylation in key regulatory regions of the Foxp3 locus.

SCFAs can indirectly affect T cells through their effects on DCs. They suppress the development of bone marrow progenitors into myeloid DCs and inhibit functional maturation of DCs in vitro. For example, C4 suppressed the maturation of bone marrow-derived DCs and production of IL-12 but increased the expression of IL-23p19. Valproic acid, a branched short-chain fatty acid and potent HDAC inhibitor that suppressed the maturation of human DCs in vitro, inhibits the upregulation of T-cell–activating molecules such as MHC II, CD80, CD86, and IL-12.

These effects are combined to create the overall tolerogenic gut environment with a strong barrier function.

2.3.1.3. Microbiota and cytokine production

Microbiota produce stimulatory signals to gut macrophages to produce interleukin-1 (IL-1). IL-1 acts on type 3 innate lymphoid cells in the intestine, producing colony-stimulating factor 2 (CSF-2). CSF-2 induces myeloid cells (including dendritic cells and macrophages) to produce immune regulatory cytokines (retinoic acid and IL-10) which support the conversion and expansion of regulatory T cells (Treg) critical for maintaining immune tolerance in the gut.

Microbiota have the capacity to produce a certain set of microbial products—gut microbiota–derived butyrate and polysaccharide A PSA (e.g., *Bacteroides fragilis*) that mediates the conversion of CD4+ T cells into Interleukin (IL)-10 producing Foxp3+ Treg cells offering immune protection. Such microbiome-derived molecule further promotes immunologic tolerance via TLR2 signaling pathway directly on Foxp3(+) Treg cells [47, 48].

The "segmented filamentous bacterium (SFB)" is another symbiotic gut commensal that is capable of inducing the appearance and activation of Th17 cells in the lamina propria, which secrete the pro-inflammatory cytokine (IL-17) and thereby enhance mucosal immune responses of the host [49].

2.3.1.4. Experimental evidences illustrated the impact of dysbiosis on the immune system and T-cell function

Multiple experimental evidences revealed that a germ-free environment is associated with a decline in neutrophil count and function [42–45]. Recognition of peptidoglycans from gut

http://dx.doi.org/10.5772/67368

microbiota by the cytosolic recognition receptor nucleotide oligomerization domain 1 (NOD1) is capable of enhancing the killing activity of marrow-derived neutrophils contributing to immune integrity. A germ-free environment was associated with impaired neutrophil phagocytic function, superoxide function, and nitric oxide generation, which could not be restored upon pathogen exposure. Germ-free rats lack the microbe-derived ATP capable of stimulating dendritic cells (CD70 and CX3CR1) involved in the subsequent differentiation of Th17 cells. Additionally, in germ-free rats, systemic, not gut macrophages, were reduced, and gut macrophages lack macrophage-activation markers, such as MHC class II.

Early-life microbial exposures alter sex hormone levels and modify the progression to autoimmunity in the nonobese diabetic (NOD) mouse model of type 1 diabetes (T1D). Colonization by commensal microbes elevated serum testosterone and protected NOD males from T1D. Furthermore, transfer of gut microbiota from adult males to immature females altered the recipient's microbiota, resulting in elevated testosterone and metabolomic changes, reduced islet inflammation and autoantibody production, and T1D protection [45].

3. The gut-microbiome checkpoints

Under normal conditions the human body has established a number of locally protective mechanisms and checkpoints to maintain immune integrity. These checkpoints include:

3.1. Mucosal buffer zone: "first-line defense"

Mucosal buffer zone represents an effective physicochemical barrier which is composed of the thick mucus layer, a number of antimicrobial proteins, and secretory IgA antibodies. The components of this barrier coalesce to minimize the contact and dilute any possible pathological microbial trigger between the commensal microbes in the gut lumen and intestinal epithelial cells that line the gut wall [50, 51].

3.2. Intestinal epithelial cells: "second-line defense"

Microbiota that escape the initial "buffer zone" encounter a second defense strategy represented by the tight junctions formed between the intestinal epithelial cells featuring a physical barrier.

Epithelial cells produce a variety of antimicrobial/bactericidal proteins, such as defensins, cathelicidins, and C-type lectins and express Toll-like receptors (TLRs) in their cell membrane. Toll-like receptors (TLRs) present on the surface of cells of innate immunity recognize pathogen-associated molecular patterns (PAMPs) with activation of the signaling adaptor molecule MyD88 (myeloid differentiation primary-response protein 88) provoking a downstream inflammatory responses. Lipopolysaccharides (LPS) are important components of the outer membrane of all Gram-negative bacteria. TLR4 is a natural ligand for LPS and upon binding to LPS leads to activation of cell and secretion of inflammatory cytokines. Cytokines in turn activate cells of the adaptive immune system that generates antigen-specific response [52].

3.3. The Innate and Adaptive Immune responses of the Lamina Propria "Third-Line Defense"

The composition and function of the gut microbiota play a critical role in regulating the Th17/Treg cell balance in the lamina propria. The innate cells in lamina propria constitute an important local line of immune defense that constantly surveys the gut lumen tracing undesirable antigens. The first is the intestinal macrophage system that phagocytoses microorganisms bypassing the first- and second-line barriers. The second is the lamina propria dendritic cells (DCs, antigen-presenting cells) that present foreign peptides complexed with MHC class II molecules for priming of antigen-specific B- or T-cell receptors to initiate an adaptive immune response.

T helper cells feature another key player when primed via a complex network of receptors, cytokines, and transcription factors enabling their differentiation into several pro-inflammatory or anti-inflammatory subsets. The type 1 T helper (Th1) response develops in response to intracellular pathogens, while type 2 T helper (Th2) and type 17 T helper (Th17) cells are predominantly stimulated after identification of extracellular organisms [53, 54].

4. Dysbiosis and autoimmune inflammatory arthritis

Multiple animal models of human autoimmune diseases (AD) suggest the direct involvement of commensal microbiota in disease development. A change to a single bacterial species and/or the entire community leads to an imbalance between the pathobiome and the symbiome immune responses with breakdown of self-immune tolerance provoking a number of ADs [47]. Mono-colonization with *Lactobacillus bifidus* in IL-1 receptor antagonist knockout mice resulted in rapid onset of arthritis which was dependent on Toll-like receptor activation by *L. bifidus*. The arthritis onset was preventable by promoting a germ-free environment [52]. Mono-colonization of germ-free mouse with single gut-microbiome "segmented filamentous bacterium (SFB)" is sufficient to induce fully functional TH17 cells that produce pro-inflammatory cytokines IL-17 and drive the onset of arthritis. The SFB upregulates the production of acute-phase isoforms of serum amyloid A (SAA) in the ileum, which can act on dendritic cells (DCs) from the small intestinal lamina propria to induce Th17 differentiation [49, 55]. Also, colonization of the mice gut with *Prevotella copri* (*P. copri*) can enhance experimental dextran sulfate sodium-induced colitis which is capable of initiating a pro-inflammatory drive in human arthritis. The *P. copri* genome encodes phosphoadenosine phosphosulfate reductase, an oxidoreductase that participates in the production of thioredoxin. Thioredoxin (TRX) is a cellular reducing catalyst induced by oxidative stress and is involved in the redox regulation of transcription factors such as NF-kappa B. TRX has been widely implicated in the pathogenesis of RA with significantly increased concentrations observed in both RA serum and synovial fluid [56–58].

Finally, commensal bacteria can produce and secrete large amounts of adenosine 51-triphosphate (ATP) that can activate a unique subset of lamina propria cells, CD70highCD11clow cells. The CD70highCD11clow subset cells could express Th17-inducing molecules, such as IL-6, IL-23p19, and transforming-growth-factor-_-activating integrin AV, and induce Th17 differentiation [59].

http://dx.doi.org/10.5772/67368

The metabolome theory: The analysis of bacterial metabolites and their association with specific taxa unveiled significant scientific data on potential mechanistic link in RA. The abundance of the *Collinsella* genus correlated strongly with high levels of three metabolites (beta-alanine, alpha-aminoadipic acid, and asparagine) in RA. The immune-stimulatory role of the *Collinsella* in RA was confirmed using a human epithelial cell line and a humanized mouse model of collagen-induced arthritis (CIA). *Collinsella* increased gut permeability by reducing the expression of tight junction protein in the human intestinal epithelial cell line CACO-2, induced production of the pro-inflammatory cytokine interleukin IL-17A. In humanized CIA, *Collinsella* enhanced disease severity. All together, these data suggest that it seems to have an essential role in altering gut permeability and disease severity as confirmed in experimental arthritis [60].

5. Altered Gut Microbiota and Inflammation in Rheumatoid Arthritis.

The Th17 pathway is one of the main inflammatory pathways. Th17 cells and its signature cytokine IL-17 have been involved in mediating pannus growth, osteoclastogenesis, and synovial neo-angiogenesis. Circulating Th17 cells as well as the IL-17 are significantly elevated in patients with RA. IL-17 induces RANKL expression in human synovial fibroblasts, leading to the loss of the RANKL/OPG balance with subsequent enhancement of osteoclastogenesis and bone erosion. IL-17 also increases the production of vascular endothelial growth factor (VEGF) in rheumatoid fibroblast-like synoviocytes (FLS), contributing to the angiogenesis in rheumatoid synovium. Finally, IL-17 stimulates the expression of various pro-inflammatory cytokines (e.g., IL-1β, TNF-α, and IL-6) and matrix-degrading enzymes (e.g., matrix metalloproteinase (MMP)-1, matrix metalloproteinase-2, matrix metalloproteinase-9, and matrix metalloproteinase-13) in whole synovial tissue, synovial fibroblasts, and cartilage, thus promoting inflammation, extracellular matrix breakdown, and cartilage destruction during RA development [61–65].

The gut mucosa represents a strategic landscape promoting a variety of interactions between the environment and the human host. They possess the potential to trigger autoimmunity in diverse ways. When genetic and/or environmental factors alter the balance in the microbiota composition, dysbiosis ensues. The metagenomics shotgun sequencing technique has revealed significant alterations in the microbiota profile in patients with RA. Evidences illustrated that changes in the symbiotic relationship between intestinal microflora and opportunistic bacteria as well as bacterial translocation from the gut to nasal mucosa or urinary tract may additionally enhance the risk of developing RA as well as disease-related comorbid conditions. Partial depletion of natural gut flora by antibiotic in experimental animals aggravates CIA [53].

Potentially harmful microorganisms/pathobiomes (such as SFB or *Lactobacillus*) dominate and create a local pro-inflammatory profile with local expansion of autoreactive Th1 and Th17-cell compartments, via secretion of stimulatory molecules as ATP adenosine-5′-triphosphate, SAA serum amyloid A, or CCL5 CC-chemokine ligand 5 signaling. The autoreactive T cells migrate to peripheral immune compartments and activate B cells to differentiate into autoantibody-producing plasma cells. These cells and antibodies then migrate to synovial tissue where the inflammatory cascade is amplified through the activation of effector components, including macrophages, fibroblasts, osteoclasts, cytokines, and proteinases provoking arthritis and pannus formation. Dysbiosis in RA is associated with clinical indices of immune-mediated inflammation, such as the titers of immunoglobulin, autoantibodies, anti-cyclic citrullinated peptide (anti-CCP), and rheumatoid factor (RF) [17, 52, 55, 66].

5.1. Microbial colonies overpresented in RA

5.1.1. The Lactobacillus species

Lactobacillus fecal microbiome communities were found to be significantly increased in patients with early RA with those from healthy individuals [25] (**Table 1**). The abundance of *Lactobacillus salivarius* was associated with an increase in disease severity associating the increase in bacterial load.

Study	Patients vs. controls (number)	Sample	Technique	Microbiota profile Increased (++), decreased (--)
Vaahtovuo et al. [67]	Early RA (n= 51) vs. fibromyalgia (n= 50)	Stool	16S rRNA hybridization and DNA staining	Bifidobacteria --, *Bacteroides* --, Porphyromonas --, *Prevotella* --, *Bacteroides fragilis* --, *Clostridium coccoides* --
Gul'neva et al. [68]	Treatment-naïve RA (n= 94) vs. healthy (n= 97)	Stool, dental, saliva	Metagenomic shotgun sequencing	*Lactobacillus salivarius* ++, *Gordonibacter pamelaeae* ++, *Clostridium asparagiforme* ++, *Haemophilus* spp. --
Liu et al. [69]	Early RA (n= 15) vs. healthy (n= 15)	Stool	Quantitative real-time PCR	*Lactobacillus* ++
Scher et al. [57]	New-onset RA (n= 44) vs. healthy (n= 28)	Stool	16S rRNA gene and WGS sequencing	Prevotella copri ++, Bacteroidetes --
Zhang et al. [70]	RA (n= 30) vs. healthy (n= 30)	Stool	16S rRNA gene and WGS sequencing	Enterococci ++, Clostridia ++, Colibacteria ++, Lactobacteria --

Table 1. Microbiota profile in RA [57, 67–70].

5.1.2. The Prevotella copri species

A strong positive correlation was illustrated between the *Prevotella copri* (*P. copri*) and new-onset untreated RA (NORA). *Prevotella* was found to be overrepresented in NORA patients, and the relative abundance of *P. copri* in RA patients negatively correlates with the presence of HLA-DRB1-shared epitope. The relation between this specific microbiome and RA was further confirmed by the observation that the expansion of *P. copri* in RA patients could be suppressed to a similar state that was observed in healthy subjects after treatment with DMARDs that control of RA disease activity.

5.1.3. Other forms of gut microbiota

RA patients showed a dysbiotic gut microbiota characterized by a decrease in *Faecalibacterium* and an increase in *Collinsella* and *Eggerthella*. Large microbiota clusters including *Gordonibacter pamelaeae, Clostridium asparagiforme, Eggerthella lenta,* and Lachnospiraceae bacterium as well as small clusters of *Bifidobacterium dentium* and *Ruminococcus lactaris* were enriched in the gut of RA patients.

On the other hand, RA patients have significantly less bifidobacteria and microbiome of the *Bacteroides-Porphyromonas-Prevotella* group, *Bacteroides fragilis* subgroup, and *Eubacterium rectale-Clostridium coccoides* group and *Haemophilus* spp. in comparison to patients with non-inflammatory rheumatic diseases.

5.1.4. Protective microbiota species: Prevotella histicola "P. histicola"

Oral feeding of *P. histicola* in mouse models of RA led to decreased symptom frequency and severity and fewer signs of inflammation in diseased vs. controls. *P. histicola* administration is associated with an upregulation of the anti-inflammatory cytokine IL-10 and Treg cells in the lamina propria and spleen of mice with CIA with subsequent amelioration of immune inflammatory responses. *P. histicola* preserves gut epithelium integrity by lowering gut permeability and increased expression of tight junction proteins (zonulin and occludin) in treated mice compared to control. Treatment with *P. histicola* had fewer side effects (such as weight gain, villous atrophy, and increased gut permeability) that are linked with nonsteroidal anti-inflammatory drugs and other traditional medications used for treating RA. This microbiome is currently considered as potential future novel therapy in RA [71].

6. Future perspectives

Multiple lines of evidence support the potential pathogenic role of gut dysbiosis in RA which makes gut microbiota a possibly promising new territory for drug targeting [72]. Restoring balance of gut microbiota might contribute to the improvement of disease symptoms in RA. Experimental models demonstrated the ability of certain microbial colonies to drive inflammation such as *P. copri* and SFB.

Thus, it is plausible to hypothesize that targeting the postulated pathobiomes might contribute to clinical improvement in RA. Despite the successful use of antimicrobials in RA, they lack microbial specificity in most studies.

"Mapping of the individual's microbiota profile and tracking their metabolic signatures might serve in the future design of a predictive profile of the potential to develop inflammatory arthritis, anticipate disease course, severity and specify more therapeutic strategies."

"Restoring balance in dysbiosis represents an advent toward novel treat to target therapeutic strategies in RA, a promising step toward an effective personalized medical approach."

Author details

Reem Hamdy A. Mohammed[1,*] and Hesham Ibrahim I. Elmakhzangy[2]

*Address all correspondence to: rmhamdy@yahoo.com

1 Department of Rheumatology/Clinical Immunology and Rehabilitation, School of Medicine, Cairo University-FRCP, Egypt

2 Department of Gastroenterology/Hepatology and Tropical Medicine, School of Medicine, Cairo University, Egypt

References

[1] Gregersen PK, Silver J, Winchester RJ. The shared epitope hypothesis. An approach to understanding the molecular genetics of susceptibility to rheumatoid arthritis. Arthritis Rheum. 1987;30:1205–13.

[2] Wellcome Trust Case Control Consortium. Genome-wide association study of 14,000 cases of seven common diseases and 3,000 shared controls. Nature. 2007;447:661–78.

[3] Taneja V. Arthritis susceptibility and the Gut Microbiome. FEBS Lett. 2014;588(22): 4244-4249.

[4] Alauzet C, Mory F, Carlier JP, Marchandin H, Jumas-Bilak E, Lozniewski A. *Prevotella nanceiensis* sp. nov., isolated from human clinical samples. Int. J. Syst. Evolut. Microbiol. 2007;57:2216–2220.

[5] de Pablo P, Dietrich T, McAlindon TE. Association of periodontal disease and tooth loss with rheumatoid arthritis in the US population. J. Rheumatol. 2008;35:70–76.

[6] Bannatyne G, Wohlmann A. Rheumatoid arthritis: its clinical history, etiology, and pathology. Lancet. 1896; 147 (3791):1120–5.

[7] Human Microbiome Project Consortium, Huttenhower C, Gevers D, Knight R, Abubucker S, Badger JH, et al. Structure, function and diversity of the healthy human microbiome. Nature. 2012; 486 (7402):207–14.

[8] Pineda MLA, Thompson SF, Summers K, de Leon F, Pope J, Reid G. A randomized, double-blinded, placebo-controlled pilot study of probiotics in active rheumatoid arthritis. Med. Sci. Monitor. 2011;17(6):CR347–5.

[9] Moen K, Brun JG, Valen M, Skartveit L, Eribe EK, Olsen I, et al. Synovial inflammation in active rheumatoid arthritis and psoriatic arthritis facilitates trapping of a variety of oral bacterial DNAs. Clin. Exp. Rheumatol. 2006; 24:656–63.

[10] Hunter W. Oral sepsis as a cause of disease. Br. Med. J. 1900; 2: 215–216.

[11] Mikuls TR, et al. Antibody responses to *Porphyromonas gingivalis* (P. gingivalis) in subjects with rheumatoid arthritis and periodontitis. Int. Immunopharmacol. 2009; 9: 38–42.

[12] Hitchon CA, et al. Antibodies to *Porphyromonas gingivalis* are associated with anticitrullinated protein antibodies in patients with rheumatoid arthritis and their relatives. J. Rheumatol. 2010; 37: 1105–1112.

[13] Loyola-Rodriguez JP, Martinez-Martinez RE, Abud-Mendoza C, Patino-Marin N, Seymour GJ. Rheumatoid arthritis and the role of oral bacteria. J. Oral Microbiol. 2010; http://dx.doi.org/10.3402/jom.v2i0.5784.

[14] Rashid T, Jayakumar KS, Binder A, Ellis S, Cunningham P, Ebringer A. Rheumatoid arthritis patients have elevated antibodies to cross-reactive and non cross-reactive antigens from Proteus microbes. Clin. Exp. Rheumatol. 2007;25:259–267.

[15] Ebringer A, Rashid T, Wilson C. Rheumatoid arthritis, Proteus, anti-CCP antibodies and Karl Popper. Autoimmun. Rev. 2010; 9: 216–223.

[16] Newkirk MM, Zbar A, Baron M, Manges AR. Distinct bacterial colonization patterns of *Escherichia coli* subtypes associate with rheumatoid factor status in early inflammatory arthritis. Rheumatology (Oxford) 2010; 49:1311–1316.

[17] Scher JU, Abramson SB. The microbiome and rheumatoid arthritis. Nat. Rev. Rheumatol. 2011; 7: 569–578.

[18] Svartz, N. The primary cause of rheumatoid arthritis is an infection—the infectious agent exists in milk. Acta Med. Scand. 1972; 192, 231–239.

[19] Hannonen P, Mottonen T, Hakola M, Oka M. Sulfasalazine in early rheumatoid arthritis. A 48-week double-blind, prospective, placebo-controlled study. Arthritis Rheum. 1993; 36, 1501–1509.

[20] O'Dell JR, et al. Treatment of rheumatoid arthritis with methotrexate alone, sulfasalazine and hydroxychloroquine, or a combination of all three medications. N. Engl. J. Med. 1996; 334, 1287–1291.

[21] Saag KG, et al. American College of Rheumatology 2008 recommendations for the use of nonbiologic and biologic disease-modifying antirheumatic drugs in rheumatoid arthritis. Arthritis Rheum. 2008; 59, 762–784.

[22] Tilley BC, et al. Minocycline in rheumatoid arthritis. A 48-week, double-blind, placebo-controlled trial. MIRA Trial Group. Ann. Intern. Med. 1995; 122, 81–89.

[23] O'Dell JR, et al. Treatment of early seropositive rheumatoid arthritis: doxycycline plus methotrexate versus methotrexate alone. Arthritis Rheum. 2006; 54, 621–627.

[24] Saviola G, Abdi Ali L, Rossini P, Campostrini L, Coppini A, Gori M, Ianaro A, Bucci M, de Nucci G, Cirino G. Clarithromycin in rheumatoid arthritis patients not responsive to disease-modifying antirheumatic drugs: an open, uncontrolled pilot study. Clin. Exp. Rheumatol. 2002; 20: 373–378.

[25] Syer SD, Blackler RW, Martin R, de Palma G, Rossi L, Verdu E, Bercik P, Surette MG, Aucouturier A, Langella P, et al. NSAID enteropathy and bacteria: a complicated relationship. J. Gastroenterol. 2015; 50: 387–393.

[26] So JS, Kwon HK, Lee CG, Yi HJ, Park JA, Lim SY, Hwang KC, Jeon YH, Im SH. *Lactobacillus casei* suppresses experimental arthritis by down-regulating T helper 1 effector functions. Mol. Immunol. 2008; 45: 2690–2699.

[27] Smith PM, Howitt MR, Panikov N, Michaud M, Gallini CA, Bohlooly-Y M, Glickman JN, Garrett WS. The microbial metabolites, short-chain fatty acids, regulate colonic Treg cell homeostasis. Science 2013; 341: 569–573.

[28] Simon GL, Gorbach SL. Intestinal flora in health and disease. Gastroenterology. 1984;86(1):174–93.

[29] Savage DC. Microbial ecology of the gastrointestinal tract. Annu. Rev. Microbiol. 1977; 31:107–33.

[30] Yeoh N, Burton J P, Suppiah P, Reid G, Stebbings S. The role of the microbiome in rheumatic diseases. Curr. Rheumatol. Rep. 2013; 15:314.

[31] Isolauri E. Development of healthy gut microbiota early in life. J. Paediatr. Child Health. 2012; 48(3):1–6.

[32] Urbaniak C, Burton JP, Reid G. Breast, milk and microbes: a complex relationship that does not end with lactation. Women's Health (Lond Engl). 2012; 8(4):385–98.

[33] Qin J, et al. A human gut microbial gene catalogue established by metagenomic sequencing. Nature. 2010;464:59–65.

[34] Eckburg PB, et al. Diversity of the human intestinal microbial flora. Science. 2005; 308:1635–1638.

[35] Rajilić-Stojanović M, Smidt H, De Vos WM. Diversity of the human gastrointestinal tract microbiota revisited. Environ. Microbiol. 2007; 9(9):2125–2136.

[36] Van den Bogert B, De Vos WM, Zoetendal EG, Kleerebezem M. Microarray analysis and barcoded pyrosequencing provide consistent microbial profiles depending on the source of human intestinal samples. Appl. Environ. Microbiol. 2011;77(6):2071–2080.

[37] Zoetendal EG, Akkermans AD, De Vos WM. Temperature gradient gel electrophoresis analysis of 16S rRNA from human fecal samples reveals stable and host-specific communities of active bacteria. Appl. Environ. Microbiol. 1998; 64(10):3854–3859.

[38] Human Microbiome Jumpstart Reference Strains Consortium, Nelson KE, Weinstock GM, Highlander SK, Worley KC, Creasy HH, Wortman JR, Rusch DB, et al. A catalog of reference genomes from the human microbiome. Science. 2010; 328:994–999.

[39] Quigley EMM. Therapies aimed at the gut microbiota and inflammation: antibiotics, prebiotics, probiotics, synbiotics, anti-inflammatory therapies. Gastroenterol. Clin. North Am. 2011;40 (1):207–22.

[40] Dimmitt RA, Staley EM, Chuang G, Tanner SM, Soltau TD, Lorenz RG. Role of postnatal acquisition of the intestinal microbiome in the early development of immune function. J. Pediatr. Gastroenterol. Nutr. 2010; 51(3):262–73.

[41] Lerner A, Aminov R, Matthias T. Dysbiosis may trigger autoimmune diseases via inappropriate post-translational modification of host proteins. Front. Microbiol. 2016;7:84.

[42] Mortha A, Chudnovskiy A, Hashimoto D, Bogunovic M, Spencer SP, Belkaid Y, Merad M. Microbiota-dependent crosstalk between macrophages and ILC3 promotes intestinal homeostasis. Science 2014; 343: 1249-288.

[43] Aychek T and Jung S. The axis of tolerance. Science 2014; 343: 1439–1440.

[44] Furusawa Y, Obata Y, Fukuda S, Endo TA, Nakato G, Takahashi D, Nakanishi Y, Uetake C, Kato K, Kato T, et al. Commensal microbe-derived butyrate induces the differentiation of colonic regulatory T cells. Nature 2013; 504: 446–450.

[45] Markle JG, Frank DN, Mortin-Toth S, Robertson CE, Feazel LM, Rolle-Kampczyk U, von Bergen M, McCoy KD, Macpherson AJ, Danska JS. Sex differences in the gut microbiome drive hormone-dependent regulation of autoimmunity. Science 2013, 339: 1084–1088.

[46] Wu HJ, Wu E.. The role of gut microbiota in immune homeostasis and autoimmunity. Gut Microbes 2012; 3: 4–14.

[47] Kim CH, Park J, Kim M. Gut microbiota-derived short-chain fatty acids, T cells, and inflammation. Immune Network. 2014;14(6):277-288.

[48] Round JL, Lee SM, Li J, Tran G, Jabri B, Chatila TA, Mazmanian SK. The Toll-like receptor 2 pathway establishes colonization by a commensal of the human microbiota. Science 2011; 332: 974–977.

[49] Ivanov II, Atarashi K, Manel N, Brodie EL, Shima T, Karaoz U, Wei D, Goldfarb KC, Santee CA, Lynch SV, et al. Induction of intestinal Th17 cells by segmented filamentous bacteria. Cell 2009; 139: 485–498.

[50] Pullar T, Hunter JA, Capell HA. Which component of sulphasalazine is active in rheumatoid arthritis? Br. Med. J. 1985; 290: 1535–1538.

[51] Ogrendik M. Effects of clarithromycin in patients with active rheumatoid arthritis. Curr. Med. Res. Opin.2007; 23: 515–522.

[52] Abdollahi-Roodsaz S, Joosten LA, Koenders MI, Devesa I, Roelofs MF, Radstake TR, Heuvelmans-Jacobs M, Akira S, Nicklin MJ, Ribeiro-Dias F, et al. Stimulation of TLR2 and TLR4 differentially skews the balance of T cells in a mouse model of arthritis. J. Clin. Investig. 2008, 118: 205–216.

[53] Dorożyńska I, Majewska-Szczepanik M, Marcińska K, Szczepanik M. Partial depletion of natural gut flora by antibiotic aggravates collagen induced arthritis (CIA) in mice. Pharmacol. Rep. 2014; 66: 250–255.

[54] Xu J, Lian F, Zhao L, Zhao Y, Chen X, Zhang X, Guo Y, Zhang C, Zhou Q, Xue Z, et al. Structural modulation of gut microbiota during alleviation of type 2 diabetes with a Chinese herbal formula. ISME J. 2015; 9: 552–562.

[55] Wu HJ, Ivanov II, Darce J, Hattori K, Shima T, Umesaki Y, Littman DR, Benoist C, Mathis D. Gut-residing segmented filamentous bacteria drive autoimmune arthritis via T helper 17 cells. Immunity 2010; 32: 815–827.

[56] Yoshida S, Katoh T, Tetsuka T, Uno K, Matsui N, Okamoto T. Involvement of thioredoxin in rheumatoid arthritis: its costimulatory roles in the TNF-alpha-induced production of IL-6 and IL-8 from cultured synovial fibroblasts. J Immunol. 1999; 163(1):351-8

[57] Scher JU, Sczesnak A, Longman RS, Segata N, Ubeda C, Bielski C, Rostron T, Cerundolo V, Pamer EG, Abramson SB, et al. Expansion of intestinal Prevotella copri correlates with enhanced susceptibility to arthritis. Elife 2013; 2: e01202.

[58] Maurice, MM, Nakamura H, Gringhuis S, Okamoto T, Yoshida S, Kullmann F, Lechner S, van der Voort EA, Leow A, Versendaal J, et al. Expression of the thioredoxin-thioredoxin reductase system in the inflamed joints of patients with rheumatoid arthritis. Arthritis Rheum. 1999; 42: 2430–2439.

[59] Atarashi K, Nishimura J, Shima T, Umesaki Y, Yamamoto M, Onoue M, Yagita H, Ishii N, Evans R, Honda K, et al. ATP drives lamina propria T(H)17 cell differentiation. Nature 2008; 455: 808–812.

[60] Taneja V, Krco CJ, Behrens MD, Luthra HS, Griffiths MM, David CS. B cells are important as antigen presenting cells for induction of MHC-restricted arthritis in transgenic mice. Mol. Immunol. 2007; 44: 2988–2996.

[61] Lubberts E, van den Bersselaar L, Oppers-Walgreen B., Schwarzenberger P, Coenen-de Roo, CJ, Kolls JK, Joosten LA, van den Berg WB. IL-17 promotes bone erosion in murine collagen-induced arthritis through loss of the receptor activator of NF-_B ligand/osteoprotegerin balance. J. Immunol. 2003, 17, 2655–2662.

[62] Kim KW, Kim HR, Park JY, Park JS, Oh HJ, Woo YJ, Park MK, Cho ML, Lee SH. Interleukin-22 promotes osteoclastogenesis in rheumatoid arthritis through induction of RANKL in human synovial fibroblasts. Arthritis Rheum. 2012; 64: 1015–1023.

[63] Ryu S, Lee JH, Kim SI. IL-17 increased the production of vascular endothelial growth factor in rheumatoid arthritis synoviocytes. Clin. Rheumatol. 2006; 25: 16–20.

[64] Moran EM, Mullan R, McCormick J, Connolly M, Sullivan O, Fitzgerald O, Bresnihan B, Veale DJ, Fearon U. Human rheumatoid arthritis tissue production of IL-17A drives matrix and cartilage degradation: synergy with tumour necrosis factor-_Oncostatin M and response to biologic therapies. Arthritis Res. Ther. 2009; 11: R113.

[65] Jovanovic DV, Di Battista JA, Martel-Pelletier J, Jolicoeur FC, He Y, Zhang M, Mineau F, Pelletier JP. IL-17 stimulates the production and expression of proinflammatory cytokines, IL-_ and TNF-_, by human macrophages. J. Immunol. 1998; 160: 3513–3521.

[66] Catrina AI, Joshua V, Klareskog L, Malmström V. Mechanisms involved in triggering rheumatoid arthritis. Immunol. Rev. 2016; 269: 162–174.

[67] Vaahtovuo J, Munukka E, Korkeamäki M, Luukkainen R, Toivanen P. Fecal microbiota in early rheumatoid arthritis. J. Rheumatol. 2008, 35, 1500–1505.

[68] Gul'neva MIU, Noskov SM. Colonic microbial biocenosis in rheumatoid arthritis. Klin. Med. 2011; 89: 45–48.

[69] Liu X, Zou Q, Zeng B, Fang Y, Wei H. Analysis of fecal Lactobacillus community structure in patients with early rheumatoid arthritis. Curr. Microbiol. 2013; 67: 170–176.

[70] Zhang X, Zhang D, Jia H, Feng Q, Wang D, Liang D. The oral and gut microbiomes are perturbed in rheumatoid arthritis and partly normalized after treatment. Nat. Med. 2015; 21: 895–905.

[71] Jia W, Li H, Zhao L, Nicholson JK. Gut microbiota: a potential new territory for drug targeting. Nat. Rev. Drug Discov. 2008; 7: 123–129.

[72] Smith PM, Howitt MR, Panikov N, Michaud M, Gallini CA, Bohlooly-Y M, Glickman JN, Garrett WS. The microbial metabolites, short-chain fatty acids, regulate colonic Treg cell homeostasis. Science 2013; 341: 569–573.

Chapter 6

Rheumatoid Arthritis and Periodontal Disease: A Complex Interplay

Codrina Ancuta, Cristina Iordache,
Eugen Ancuta and Claudia Mihailov

Additional information is available at the end of the chapter

http://dx.doi.org/10.5772/65863

Abstract

Recent advances in understanding the dynamic pathways involved in the pathogenesis of rheumatoid arthritis have emphasized the pivotal role of pro-inflammatory cytokines, inflammatory cells, endothelial cell activation and matrix degradation, acting in a genetically predisposed environment. On the other hand, there are significant amounts of data highlighting the potential role of bacteria (leading periodonthopatic pathogen *Porfiromonas gingivalis*) in promoting different types of arthritis, as well as the influence of periodontis (an infectious-inflammatory condition) as etiological or modulating factor in different pathologies, including cardio-vascular disorders, diabetes, respiratory disease and inflammatory rheumatic disorders (such as rheumatoid arthritis, ankylosing spondylitis and lupus). The present chapter deals with the possible association between rheumatoid arthritis and periodontitis as entities with common pathological events.

Keywords: rheumatoid arthritis, periodontitis, *Porfiromonas gingivalis,* citrullination, anti-citrullinated antibodies

1. Introduction

Rheumatoid arthritis (RA) and periodontitis are chronic inflammatory disorders that share a complex, multifaceted host-mediated pathobiology promoted by significant levels of inflammatory mediators that are able to induce synovium and periodontal tissues inflammation, joint damage and alveolar bone loss, respectively [1–7].

RA, a chronic inflammatory autoimmune disease with articular as well as systemic consequences, is outlined by a dynamic pathobiology with chronic synovitis as the epicenter of immunologic responses, inflammation and tissue destruction, occurring as a response to an initiating event (microbial exposure) or a putative antigen in genetically predisposed host [1–11].

On the other hand, known as a destructive, dysbiotic inflammatory condition that concerns gums, periodontal disease or periodontitis is typically characterized by rapid tooth loss directed by local anaerobic bacterial colonization (the "red complex" microorganisms with leading *Porphiromonas gingivalis*), biofilm-related periodontal inflammation, subsequent neutrophilic and immune activation, soft tissue destruction and alveolar bone loss [1–12].

The bidirectional relationship between periodontitis and RA is governed by common genetic (HLA-DR) and environmental influences (smoking), chronic inflammatory events with immunoregulatory imbalance (excessive TNF-α, IL-1β, IL-6, IL-11, IL-17 activation, prostaglandin E2, nitric oxide, matrix metalloproteinases), osteoclast activation (RANKL overregulation) promoting active bone destruction and periodontal lesions, bacterial factors, persistence of antigens, citrullination of endogenous proteins by the means of peptidyl arginine deiminase as second inflammatory event [1–13].

Furthermore, the association among periodontal disease and RA has been extensively addressed in recent years, emphasizing the role of gingival microorganisms, particularly *Porphyromonas gingivalis* (*P. gingivalis*), as the underlying link between dental and rheumatic pathology via citrullination [1–10].

We systematically reviewed data from literature focusing on inflammation and tissue-damaging aspects, oral microbiota, antibodies against bacteria and autoantibodies and treatment for both RA and periodontitis, aiming to explore the relationship between both diseases.

2. A closer look to periodontitis

2.1. Pathobiology of periodontitis

As a chronic immuno-inflammatory disease and a consequence of an infectious trigger that originally involves gingival soft tissue, periodontitis is classically characterized by the destruction of periodontium and surrounding connective tissue matrix [1–11]. It is a complex, dynamic and progressive condition, resulting from a continuing cross-talk between microbial challenge and host inflammatory and immune response [1–7].

The extent and severity of periodontitis, as well as disease staging covers a sequence of pathobiologic steps comprising gingivitis, plaque accumulation and chronic inflammation, colonization by periodontopathogenic anaerobes, loss of connective tissue attachments to teeth, bone resorption and, ultimately, tooth loss [1–10].

The oral cavity behaves as a perpetual source of infectious, generally nonpathogenic agents; however, subgingival microbiota may accumulate to shape this biofilm through particular settings, and favor networking between pathogens and host tissues, with or without direct dissemination [1–11].

The pathways underlying chronic periodontitis encompass for an intricate array of events, starting with gingival colonization by *P. gingivalis*, chronic inflammation, immune-mediated periodontal damage and alveolar bone loss, local citrullination, host immune response [1–11].

A schematic overview of the microbial and host-associated pathology in periodontal disease is represented in **Figure 1**.

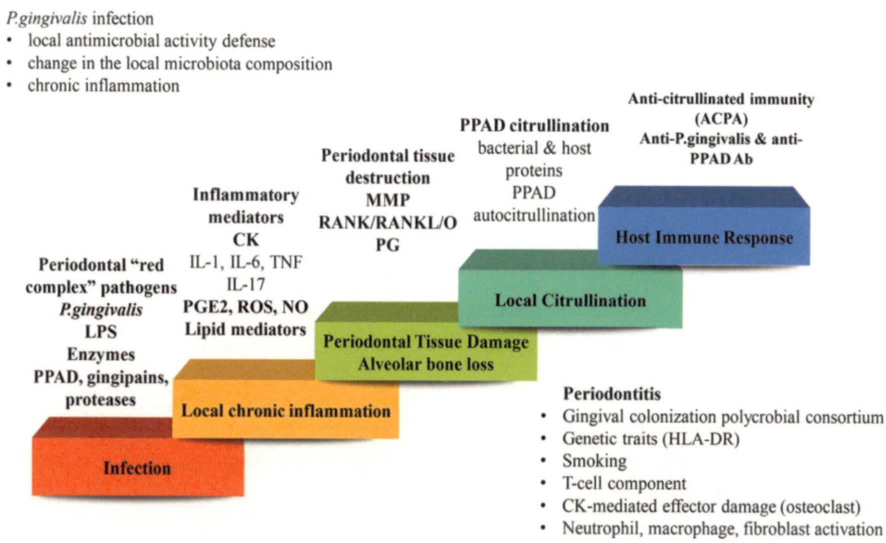

Figure 1. Sequence of events in chronic periodontitis.

It is widely recognized that the oral microbiota arising in a tolerant genetic background is involved in the initiation and extension of periodontal disease [1–12]. Several bacterial species, e.g., *P. gingivalis, Treponema denticola (T. denticola), Tannerella forsythia (T. forsythia)* and *Aggregatibacter actinomycetemcimtans*, the so-called red complex [1–12], remain of particular relevance as they are true pathogens and late colonizers of the oral biofilm, act synergistically and by co-aggregation with the support of attaching bacteria through specific adhesion molecules [1–10].

Further, *P. gingivalis* is able to release pathogen-associated molecular patterns, specifically lipopolissacharides (LPS), peptidoglycans, proteases and lytic enzymes, engaging local immune cell trafficking and activation—neutrophils (acting to protect the host from periodontal pathogens as the first-line defenders), macrophages (as potent antigen-presenting cells), T-cells and B-cells (perpetuating and amplifying inflammatory response and antibody synthesis) [1–11].

However, *P. gingivalis* escapes the local antimicrobial defense as a result of delayed neutrophil apoptosis and complement system manipulation with subsequent change in the gingival bacterial composition [11].

To better understand, *P. gingivalis* encourages the immune subversion by several strategies including: IL-8 inhibition, complement manipulation and toll-like receptor 4 (TLR4) antagonism, leading to impaired host defense. Symbiotic gingival microbiota with tissue homeostasis swaps to dysbiotic environment, with inflammation and bone loss as main attributes of periodontal disease [1, 8, 11, 12].

Locally recruited cells release a wide range of factors, such as pro-inflammatory cytokines (TNF-α, IL-1β, IL-6, IL-8, IL-12, IL-11, IL-17), reactive oxygen species, prostaglandin E2, nitric oxide, and other inflammatory mediators in the gingival tissue and gingival crevicular fluid as well [1–5, 11–14]. Otherwise, anti–inflammatory cytokines including IL-10 and TGF-β1 are down regulated in active periodontal lesions, demonstrating an imbalance between pro- and anti-inflammatory systems in the periodontal microenvironment [1, 11].

Although the initial trigger of gingival inflammation is microbial, the cytokine-mediated damage is largely host-associated [1–10]. Hence, augmented TNF-α, IL-1β, IL-6, IL-11, and, particularly, IL-17 directly control the Receptor Activator of NF-κB/Receptor Activator of NF-κB Ligand/osteoprotegerin (RANK/RANKL/OPG) system and stimulate osteoclastogenesis through increasing RANKL expression reducing OPG synthesis in osteoblasts and stromal cells [1–11, 15]. Connective tissue matrix degradation is supplementary dependent on matrix metalloproteinases (MMPs) and other proteolytic enzymes discharged by resident activated fibroblasts [1, 10, 11].

Of particular interest, *P. gingivalis*-dependent protein citrullination and the immune response to the periodontal infective aggression involving both innate and adaptive immunity (e.g., anti-citrullinated immunity and IgG anti-*P. gingivalis* antibodies) additionally outline the complexity of pathogenic pathways in periodontitis [1–5, 7–10, 15].

Periodontis is a multifactorial condition, where environmental factors (including oral hygiene, gingival bacterial plaque, smoking, stress), and genetic polymorphism (HLA-DR alleles, IL-1 gene promoter, IL-6 and IL-10 genes) perform critical role in the expression of the disease [1, 4, 10, 11, 15, 16].

Recent data agreed that chronic periodontitis is a risk factor for many multisystem diseases including rheumatoid arthritis and other auto-inflammatory rheumatic conditions, cardio and cerebrovascular disease (atherosclerosis, myocardial infarction, stroke), diabetes, osteoporosis, respiratory and neurodegenerative disorders, adverse pregnancy outcomes [1, 17, 18]. In fact, locally exacerbated and ongoing systemic inflammation, specific tissue damage, mutual triggers (smoking, iatrogenic factors) acting in a genetic vulnerable individuals (HLA-DRβ1) uphold a modulating bidirectional relationship between periodontitis and the above mentioned entities [1–18].

It is obvious that chronic periodontitis remains an authentic infection of the oral cavity; biofilm-associated specific microorganisms are essential but not sufficient, as the bacterial eradication does not spontaneously manage to resolution of periodontitis [1–18].

http://dx.doi.org/10.5772/65863

2.2. *Porphyromonas gingivalis* as a key player in periodontitis

Chronic periodontitis is, therefore, typically initiated by the colonization of dental plaque by a core set of periodontal pathogens, specifically *P. gingivalis, T. forsythia* and *T. denticola,* documented as the "red complex", prototype of polybacterial pathogenic consortium in periodontitis [1–5, 7–11, 19].

P. gingivalis, a leading microorganism in this dysbiotic setting, is a gram-negative anaerobic bacteria, involved in the onset of inflammation and tissue destruction during periodontal disease [1–11]. It is ordinarily found in small number in a healthy oral cavity [11], but the pathology occurs when *P. gingivalis* binds to and accumulates on the tooth surface, leading to the development of a mixed biofilm, the expansion of the bacteria into the gingival sulcus and the formation of a periodontal pocket [11, 19].

P. gingivalis is an outstanding example of a bacteria able to shape the periodontal microenvironment and to destabilize the homeostatic immune system endorsing chronic inflammation and tissue damage as well [11].

At least four mechanisms currently advocate for its essential role in the pathobiology of periodontal disease: (i) the release of specific virulence factors such as specific lipopolysaccharide (LPS), fimbrae, hemagglutins and several enzymes, mainly cysteine proteases (gingipains), but also collagenase, gelatinase, hyaluronidase promoting a chronic inflammatory setting and local invasion [2, 3, 11, 20]; (ii) the expression of peptidyl arginine deiminase (PAD) involved in tissue citrullination, loss of tolerance against neo-epitopes and subsequent activation of adaptive immune response [1, 2, 3, 20]; (iii) auto-citrullination of its own PAD [1, 2, 3, 11, 20]; and (iv) enable other co-aggregating pathogenic bacteria to remain in the periodontal tissue [2].

P. gingivalis expresses atypical LPS, proceeding either as a weak TLR4 agonist or even a TLR4 antagonist, enabling the colonization and invasion of periodontal pockets as it becomes immunologically silent [1, 2, 8, 11, 21]. Furthermore, *P.gingivalis* invades gingival epithelial cells via binding through its fimbriae to β1 integrin on the host epithelial cell surface [4, 5, 11] and blocks apoptosis through the PI3K/Akt and JAK/Stat pathways, allowing intracellular bacterial proliferation [11].

The true virulence of *P. gingivalis* is, however, associated with its proteolytic enzymes, particularly extracellular arginine and lysine-specific cysteine endopeptidases (gingipain R and gingipain K, respectively) [1–5, 11]. Gingipains are skilled to facilitate the evasion of host defense and cause tissue injury by activation of MMPs (1, 3, 9) and further degradation of host proteins (laminin, fibronectin and collagen) [1, 2, 8 11, 22–24]. Moreover, these enzymes are responsible for the resistance of *P. gingivalis* killing by complement [1, 2, 8, 11]. Remarkably, the degradation of microbial peptides by gingipains allows other pathogenic bacteria co-aggregating with *P. gingivalis* to persist in the gingiva [2, 8, 11, 15, 20, 25]. Finally, gingipains affect proinflammatory signaling pathways by cleavage and activation of the proteinase-activated receptor-2 on human neutrophils [2, 11, 15, 20]. Futile attempts by the host immune response to eliminate infection subsequently lead to connective tissue damage, including alveolar bone resorption [22].

P. gingivalis is a particular periodontal pathogen that expresses endogenous peptidyl-arginine deiminase (PPAD), a citrullinating enzyme bearing potential to generate antigens driving autoimmunity in susceptible individuals [1, 2, 8, 10, 11].

It is worth mentioning that the switching of a charged arginine residue to an uncharged citrulline results in evident, irreversible posttranslational protein modifications, meaning changes in the three-dimensional conformation and abnormal function [8, 10, 17]. Citrullinated antigens as neo-epitopes in the periodontal tissues may selectively activate adaptive immune response and break the self-tolerance leading to severe aggressive periodontitis, anti-cyclic citrullinated peptides, anti-*P. gingivalis* antibodies as well, and, potentially, to the development of RA in genetically predisposed hosts [1–3, 20, 25].

PAD-mediated citrullination is also responsible for evading host defense against *P. gingivalis* by two additional mechanisms: generation of ammonia that result in a favorable microenvironment for anaerobic bacteria and inactivation of certain chemokines contributing to neutrophil recruitment into the gingiva [8, 10, 11, 17].

Besides, *P. gingivalis* stimulates a true "local chemokine paralysis" by inhibiting the expression of IL-18 on epithelial cells [8, 11], delaying the traffic of neutrophils and, therefore, permitting its persistence and/or proliferation in the periodontal tissue with subsequent modification of the subgingival microbiota [11, 25].

2.3. *P. gingivalis* peptidyl-arginine deiminase (PPAD) *versus* peptidyl-arginine deiminase (PAD) biology

There is accumulating evidence to outline the citrullination status and biology of PPAD *versus* human PAD, supporting the hypothesis that PPAD is a reliable challenger for inducing autoimmunity, with particular relevance to the pathogenesis of RA [1, 2, 10, 11, 17, 20, 22, 26, 27].

This apparently distinctive bacterial enzyme is effective in generating citrullinated proteins (bacterial and human) and, furthermore, has the ability to autocitrullinate, eliciting the loss of immune tolerance and synthesis of autoantibodies in susceptible individuals [1–5, 7–11, 22].

To date, five isoforms of human PADs (PAD1, 2, 3, 4/5, and 6) are described, with specificities for different tissues and different physiological functions [2, 3, 10]; however, none of them present strict homology with bacterial PAD [1, 2, 10, 11, 17, 27], and only PAD2 and PAD4 are expressed at the synovial level and involved in RA [1, 3, 10, 26].

The main differences between human and bacterial PAD focus on the mechanism of activation and substrates undergoing citrullination [1, 10, 11]. Thus, PPAD is a calcium-independent enzyme that becomes active at higher pH that PAD; its action is facilitated by the co-localization with arginine-specific gingipains in the outer membrane of *P. gingivalis* [1, 2, 10, 11, 20, 25]. PPAD act specifically on C-terminal arginine residues and free arginine [1, 2], events enabled by the proteolytic activity of gingipains. In fact, we talk about a two-step process in the inflamed-infected periodontal sites, initiated by cysteine protease gingipains that cleave protein chains and expose the C-terminal arginine, facilitating the secondary intervention of PPAD [1, 2, 10, 11, 25].

Other substrates citrullinated by PPAD include peptides resulted from fibrinogen and α-enolase degradation by gingipains [2, 10], fibrin and vimentin, bradykinin with the potential impairment of kinin proinflammatory activity [2, 10, 20, 25], and the C-terminal arginine residue of the epidermal growth factor influencing its biologic activity [2, 10, 25, 27, 28].

Finally, PPAD allows, either directly or indirectly (via enhancement of inflammatory reactions and release of host PADs), the abnormal citrullination of bacterial and human proteins with the assembly of the so-called cryptic-epitopes and subsequent antibody production [1, 2, 10, 11, 20, 25].

2.4. PPAD and PAD autocitrullination

Although PPAD preferentially citrullinates different bacterial and/or host peptides bearing C-terminal arginine, it becomes clear that this enzyme may undergo autocitrullination and, hence, stimulate a specific pattern of autoimmunity and request for autoantibody response in permissive genetic background (carriers of HLA-DRB1 shared epitope) [2, 10, 20]. There is a heightened immune response to *P. gingivalis* and IgG specifically targeting autocitrullinated PPAD in chronic periodontal disease and rheumatoid arthritis which could perpetuate the immune response through epitope spreading and cross-reactivity with citrullinated human proteins suggesting a potential mechanistic linkage between the two disorders [10, 11, 25, 29, 30]. Of interest, PAD4 also experiences autocitrullination, and antibodies recognizing this isoform of human PAD embrace predictive value in RA [10, 11, 26, 27, 31].

To summarize, the infection with *P. gingivalis* triggers a broad spectrum of local and systemic inflammatory, destructive and immune events in susceptible individuals. Strategic steps in the complex pathobiology of periodontitis comprise early release of a true arsenal of specialized virulence factors and bacteria-danger signals (LPS, fimbriae, peptidoglycan, various proteolytic enzymes) exerting both direct and indirect effects (via stimulation of inflammatory and immune pathways, release of host PAD), followed by aberrant PPAD-dependent citrullination of different substrates such as host-derived and bacterial proteins, as well as PPAD-autocitrullination, with subsequent generation of criptic epitopes and autoantibody synthesis. Finally, the immune subversion endorses loss of tolerance to structurally similar host proteins and outcomes the induction of anti-cyclic citrullinated antibodies suggesting the relationship between chronic periodontitis and rheumatoid arthritis [1, 2, 10, 13, 17, 19, 20, 25].

3. Role of citrullination in rheumatoid arthritis development

Citrullination is a posttranslational modification of proteins at arginine residues reported in a wide range of tissues and settings, holding relevant physiologic as well as pathologic implications [10, 17, 27, 32]. Although considered a critical event in different inflammatory conditions, currently available data emphasize the link between citrullination and autoimmune diseases, suggesting that immunity towards citrullinated self-proteins rather than citrullination itself is a specific event in RA [10, 17, 27].

3.1. Citrullination and inflammation

Abnormal citrullination of endogenous proteins is typically acknowledged as an initial, tactical process in the complex pathobiology of RA, driving the induction of altered self-epitopes and extensive autoimmune response [10, 17, 27].

Moreover, immunogenicity of these new antigens explains the presence of antibodies against citrullinated peptides (ACPA) considered not only diagnostic biomarkers for RA and prognostic factors for severe aggressive disease, but also consuming a pathogenic role [10, 17, 27]. Nevertheless, only individuals with definite HLA polymorphisms, such as the conserved region of HLA-DRB1 alleles are at risk to recognize as "nonself" such citrullinated proteins and to develop RA [1, 2, 10, 17, 27].

Along with glycosylation and carbamylation, citrullination is basically involved in many physiological processes in a variety of tissues, biochemical enzymatic reactions leading to structural and functional protein/peptide modification [2, 10, 17, 27]. Conversely, dysfunctional posttranslational protein modifications are often reported during autoinflammatory pathology, particularly RA, evading the immunological tolerance and stimulating a specific profile of humoral response [2, 10, 17, 26, 27].

As mentioned before, citrullination or deamination strictly encompass for a change of arginine with citrulline, meaning that an imine nitrogen of arginine-residues is replaced by an atom of oxygen; accordingly, histone modification, genomic regulation and neutrophils extracellular trap (NET) formation are described and engaged in development of newly citrullinated antigens [10, 17, 27].

It is well-known that citrullination constantly requires the activation and intervention of PAD-family enzymes at intra and/or extracellular levels in a Ca^{2+}-dependent manner, and only two out of the five human PAD subtypes (PAD 2 and PAD4) are relevant for RA based on their expression in joints, immune cells, neutrophils and mast cells [1, 10, 11, 12, 17, 26, 27]. Thus, PAD-mediated citrullination could be easily classified as a basic cellular damage but also an inflammatory process occurring in a range of inflammatory backgrounds such as synovial tissue, gingival and periodontal sites and lungs, challenging local immunity [10, 17, 27].

On the other hand, recent advances in understanding the pathophysiology of chronic periodontal infection with *P. gingivalis*, and the potential connection between periodontitis and systemic disorders including RA, have reemphasized the role of this periodonthopathic microbe as one of the risk factors for RA in a permissive genetic context [1–11, 17, 27].

P. gingivalis is the only known periodontal bacteria in the gingival microbiota that expresses a PPAD able to initiate and perpetuate a gradual autoimmune process through epitope-spreading by peptide citrullination (bacterial, PPAD itself as a citrulllinated bacterial protein), cross-reactivity with citrullinated human proteins and ACPA synthesis [1, 2, 10, 11, 25].

The break of tolerance to one citrullinated epitope predisposes to break of tolerance to additional citrullinated epitopes; the initial mechanism might be more related to recognition of citrullinated antigen per se than to a particular citrullinated autoantigen [10, 11, 26, 32, 33].

3.2. Smoking, citrullination and rheumatoid arthritis

Environment-triggered citrullination (smoking, bacterial infections) in articular and extra-articular locations essentially progress to specific immunity and disease in genetic predisposed individuals [1, 2, 10, 12, 16, 32, 34, 35]. Smoking is a well-known risk factor for RA, particularly, in ACPA-positive subsets. Cigarette smoking leads to a sequence of events responsible for local increase in PAD enzyme expression and consequent generation of protein citrullination in the lung [10, 12, 17, 27]. Chronic exposure to self-citrullinated epitopes could further contribute to the loss of immune tolerance and gradual occurrence of humoral immune response towards some of the citrullinated autoantigens (ACPA) [10, 17, 27]. However, smoking and other risk factors might lead to breaking of immune tolerance only in the presence of genetic risk factors for ACPA positive RA [10, 12, 17, 26, 27, 36].

3.3. Anti-citrullinated proteins/peptide antibodies (ACPA) pathobiology

ACPAs, the autoimmune signature of RA, are sensitive and specific diagnostic, prognostic and therapeutic biomarkers in RA; they are detected from very early phases of the disease, up to a decade prior to the RA clinical onset, and feature a dynamic correlation with RA severity, clinical outcomes and efficacy of synthetic and biologic therapies [10, 37, 38]. In fact, ACPAs are a family of partly cross-reactive antibodies which target citrullinated self-proteins and peptides abundant in inflamed joints, such as fibrinogen, fibronectin, vimentin and vinculin, β-enolase, histone, biglycan, clusterin, collagen type II, keratin. So far, 53 such citrullinated members are identified, an assembly called "citrullinome" [10, 12, 17, 27].

According to the ACPA status, RA could be classified in two distinct clinical phenotypes with particular genetics, risk factors, immunopathology, clinical and treatment outcomes; thus, ACPA-positive RA is defined by a specific genetic (HLA-DRB1*0401 and *0404)- environmental interface (e.g., smoking and *P. gingivalis* infection), higher disease severity (erosive RA, extra-articular involvement, comorbidities) and poor remission rates. Besides, high ACPA titers could predict clinical response with B-cell depletive agents (rituximab) or selective co-stimulation modulators (abatacept), independently of disease activity and, therefore, might help to define therapeutic RA profiles [10, 11, 16, 17, 27, 28, 36].

Interestingly, ACPA specificities may also account for distinctive clinical RA subtypes: anti-citrullinated vimentin antibodies may be better prognostic factors for radiographic progression, while anti-citrullinated enolase antibodies predict clinical outcomes [10, 17, 27].

ACPAs are detected as antibodies against cyclic citrullinated proteins (anti-CCP antibodies) which are detectable by specific assays in RA patients, and their screening performance largely varies with different tests: sensitivity and specificity significantly improved with third-generation assays, as well as the ability to identify those subjects with undifferentiated arthritis who are likely to develop RA [10, 17]. Conversely, second-generation tests are classically more specific for longstanding, established disease [10, 17, 39].

The exact molecular pathways of anti-citrullinated immunity in RA are still obscure, but it is clear that ACPAs encourage the perpetuation of synovial inflammation via binding to citrullinated proteins positioned in the cellular membrane, attached to a variety of cellular receptors (such as TLR4 or FcγR) or incorporated in NETs [1–4, 10, 11, 17]. Furthermore, complement binding and activation may enhance local inflammation [7, 12, 17, 27].

ACPAs are constantly produced in the inflamed synovial microenvironment by locally activated B cells [17, 27] and stimulate TNFα production, as well as direct bone injury by osteoclast activation [6, 10, 17, 27, 39, 40].

Overall, the effector functions of different well-defined ACPA may adjust according to antibody specificities. Thus, reactivity towards citrullinated vimentin as well as anti-cartilage-specific protein collagen II antibodies directly bind to osteoclast surface and modulate their activation, determining subchondral bone erosive lesions and osteoporosis [10, 12, 40]. On the other hand, antibodies to autoantigenic enolase and histones focus on local inflammation [10, 12, 17, 27], as ACPAs are able to induce NETs.

3.4. The paradigm of citrullination and ACPA in the development of ACPA positive rheumatoid arthritis

The environmental exposure (such as smoking, silica and other nanomaterials of air pollution, bacterial infection, e.g., *P. gingivalis*) and the genetic determinants (MHC class II alleles) enable abnormal citrullination and support immunity against citrullinated proteins in certain extra-articular sites (lung, periodontal tissue). The relationship between the emergence of local ACPAs as the first sign of autoimmunity and RA is further supported by the documentation of shared citrullinated peptides in the lungs, periodontal sites and joints as potential ACPA epitope bearing proteins [10, 17, 27].

A second event might promote aberrant synovial citrullination, local impaired immunity, generation of ACPA for several immune-dominant citrullinated peptide, chronic inflammation and tissue-specific damage [10, 17, 27].

4. The biological link between periodontitis and rheumatoid arthritis

Continuing periodontal disease as a trigger for chronic arthritis in susceptible individuals via dysregulation in oral microbiota and host immune barriers is a reliable, but still debatable concept [1, 2, 8, 10–12]. The old paradigm indicates that RA could be a consistent risk factor for chronic periodontitis: impaired periodontal health labels the multifactorial and synergistic result of compromised joint functionality (hand as well as temporomandibular joint), oral dryness (secondary Sjogren's) and specific RA medications [8].

In contrast, newer theories emphasize that periodontal disease is a risk factor for RA: both are multifaceted disorders with shared pathogenic mechanisms such as local and systemic excess of inflammation, irreversible bone injury, aberrant activation of the immune system with an extra dose of autoimmunity and a common genetic background [1–5, 8, 41–45].

4.1. Evidences relating periodontitis and rheumatoid arthritis

Substantial amount of research trying to clarify the potential relationship between RA and periodontitis was published during the last decade [1–13]. Nevertheless, the true prevalence, causality, significance, related factors (e.g., smoking habits, oral hygiene, ACPA positivity), together with therapeutic intervention (periodontal host modulation therapy, synthetic remissive drugs, biologics) to mitigate both RA and periodontal disease are still controversial [1–13, 17, 27].

Overwhelming evidence coming from cross-sectional studies [1–13, 10, 40, 46–48] showed a statistically significant correlation between RA and periodontitis (prevalence and/or severity); nevertheless, other cohort-based or case-control studies noticed no association between oral health and rheumatic inflammatory pathology [1, 2, 10, 12]. The conflicting reports may be explained by differences between study populations, sample size, adjustments for confounders (age, gender, race/ethnicity, smoking status, RA activity and medication) and lack of uniformity in disease classification criteria for periodontal disease [49].

The probability of periodontitis among RA is higher compared to healthy individuals [1–4, 8, 47], while the severity greater [1–4, 8, 15, 47], meaning that subjects diagnosed with RA experience more periodontal disease and more periodontal destruction [1, 8, 15]. Furthermore, moderate to severe periodontitis is characteristically described in different settings of RA [1, 8], and vice-versa, higher RA prevalence among patients with advanced periodontitis [1, 8, 15, 47, 49]. Both early and established RA are characterized by substantial periodontal disease compared with presumably healthy non-RA controls [1–4, 6, 8, 44, 45]: higher prevalence of self-reported periodontal symptoms [8], significant more gingival bleeding on probing [1–4, 6, 8], a greater number of missing teeth [1–4, 6, 8], deeper periodontal pockets [1–4, 6, 8], more clinical attachment loss [1–4, 6, 8] and increased alveolar bone injury [1–4, 6, 8] versus healthy controls with comparable oral hygiene [1–4, 6, 8, 44, 45].

More specifically, a meaningful positive correlation between measures of RA activity and extent and severity of periodontitis was reported: high disease activity (DAS28 scores) is generally demonstrated in RA with aggressive periodontitis as compared to RA without or with moderate periodontitis, even after adjusting for multiple confounders [4, 8, 47].

A systematic review of cross-sectional trials further strengthens the evidence addressing periodontitis in relation to autoimmunity damage in RA. Overall, significantly higher ACPA, rheumatoid factor and antibodies to *P. gingivalis* were described among RA with periodontitis than those without periodontal disease [4, 8, 11, 47], whereas increased alveolar bone loss was significantly associated with ACPA positivity in the same patient population [4]. Similarly, detailed analysis of ACPA specificities (citrullinated vimentin and histone) showed increased levels in RA associated with both moderate and high alveolar loss, without differences based on smoking status [4, 15, 16, 26, 48–50]. It seems that periodontitis is a strong predictor of ACPA positivity in RA [8], whereas IgG and IgM ACPA subtypes are highly associated with antibodies against *P. gingivalis* [2, 3, 8, 29]. Additionally, in refractory RA with periodontitis the most powerful anaerobes identified in synovial fluid are *P. intermedia, P. gingivalis* and *T. denticola* [1, 40, 41]. However, no difference in ACPA or rheumatoid factor levels for RA participants with mild periodontal lesions as compared to moderate or severe periodontitis were found among other studies, suggesting that ACPA status might not influence the prevalence and severity of periodontal disease [1, 8, 11, 49].

Regarding smoking as a risk factor for both conditions, subgroup analysis showed an association between RA and periodontitis irrespective to smoking behavior [4, 6, 8, 15, 16, 48, 49]; increased risk of periodontitis was demonstrated in nonsmoking RA [1, 6, 8, 11].

In particular, only a small number of studies focused on periodontitis as a primary event, occurring before clinical onset of RA *versus* periodontitis as comorbidity, described after the diagnosis of rheumatic condition [1, 8, 11].

Finally, effective treatment strategies for periodontal disease (e.g., nonsurgical treatment) on RA activity and systemic inflammation are commonly reported [1, 3, 4, 50, 51].

4.2. A parallel between chronic periodontal disease and rheumatoid arthritis

Exploring the association between chronic periodontal disease and RA has demonstrated striking similar immunological, biological and genetic underlying processes [1, 2, 4, 12, 22], although apparently totally different etiologies (autoimmune RA, infective periodontitis respectively) [10]. **Figure 2** offers a detailed synopsis of similarities between RA and periodontitis.

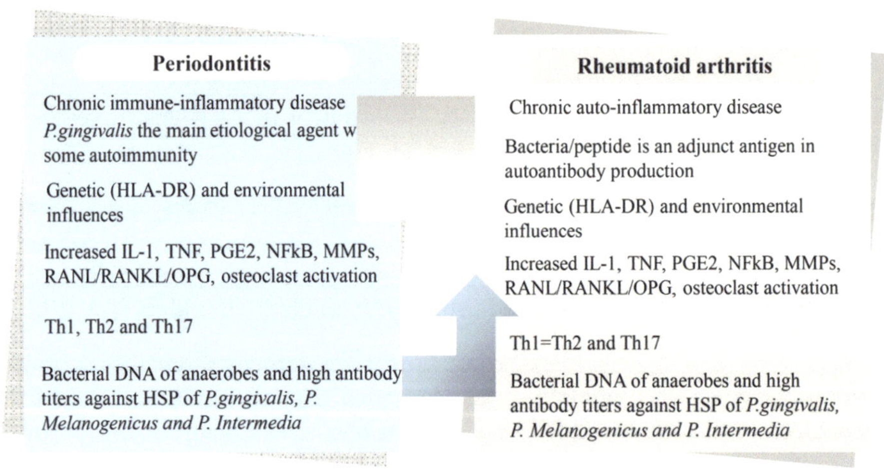

Figure 2. Similarities between PD and RA pathobiology.

Both are complex multifactorial disorders, characterized not only by a dysfunction of basic inflammatory and tissue destructive mechanisms, but also by an altered adaptive and innate immune response in individuals at risk (genetic traits) [1, 2, 8, 10, 12, 22].

The excess of local (periodontal tissue and gingival crevicular fluid in periodontitis, synovial microenvironment in RA) along with systemic chronic inflammation is driven by an imbalance between pro-inflammatory and anti-inflammatory cytokines, with persistent up-regulated pro-inflammatory signaling pathways (mainly IL-1, IL-6, TNFα, NF-kB) and higher amounts of inflammatory mediators including reactive oxygen species, nitric oxide and lipid mediators [1–3, 8, 10–12, 22]. In addition, altered connective tissue and bone homeostasis with irreversible damage of collagen-rich structures (gingiva, periodontal ligament and alveolar bone in periodontitis, subchondral bone and cartilage in RA) is essentially related to augmented activity of collagenolytic matrix metalloproteinases and other enzymes (elastase, bacterial cysteine proteases, neutrophil associated enzymes), but also to overexpression of the RANK/RANKL/OPG system [1–3, 8, 10, 12, 13, 45].

The validity of the relationship between periodontitis and RA is, furthermore, supported by a particular genetic predisposition and related environmental risk factors (e.g., smoking) [1, 8, 10, 12]; both entities share a common genetic profile (shared epitope HLA-DRB1 alleles) [1, 10, 12], while polymorphism of genes encoding inflammatory cytokines as well as IL-1 combined risk alleles which may cause a synergistic effect on bone destruction in joints and the periodontium might also confer susceptibility for RA and periodontitis [1, 8, 10, 12, 15, 16].

Finally, abnormal PAD and PPAD-mediated citrullination of the synovial and host periodontium peptides/proteins (vimentin, keratin, α-enolase), respectively, with sequential loss of tolerance against neo-epitopes account for altered local and systemic immune reactions in susceptible patients with either periodontitis or RA; the generation of citrullinated new autoantigens and patterns of antibody response by ACPA, anti-autocitrullinated PPAD, anti-autocitrullinated PAD4 and anti-heat shock proteins of *P. gingivalis* (anti-hsp70) antibodies are frequently encountered in both RA and periodontitis [1, 10, 12, 15, 25, 30, 45].

Overall, gingival citrullination and local induction of ACPA, as well as cross-reactivity between antibodies to *P. gingivalis* and ACPA may explain the link periodontitis—RA [1, 10, 12, 27].

4.3. Hypothetical model of biological link Between rheumatoid arthritis and periodontitis

A potential scenario exploring the relation between periodontitis and RA could be depicted as follows:

- oral infection with *P. gingivalis* may induce a Th17 polarization with subsequent activation of Th17 signaling pathway, synthesis of pro-inflammatory cytokines (preferentially IL-1β, IL-6, IL-22, TNF-α, TGFβ and IL-23), expression of PPAD with atypical PPAD- and PAD-dependent citrullination of gingival proteins, bacterial peptides and PPAD as well, synthesis of specific antibodies such as ACPA, anti-citrullinated PPAD and anti-*P. gingivalis* antibodies [1, 4, 8, 10–13, 19, 52];

- periodontopathic microbial biofilm and its metabolic products (lipopolysaccharides, matrix degrading enzymes and endotoxins) originally stimulate a localized inflammatory-destructive response branded by augmented levels of tissue destructive proteinases (MMP 8, 9, 13 and neutrophil elastase) and RANK/RANKL/OPG system, as well as resident cells activation (osteoclasts, fibroblasts) [1, 4, 8, 12];

- systemic inflammation and immune dysregulation particularly autoimmunity targeting self-citrullinated synovial peptides delineate one of the first events in RA [1, 4, 8, 10, 12].

Figure 3 presents the paradigm of RA—periodontitis pathogenic link.

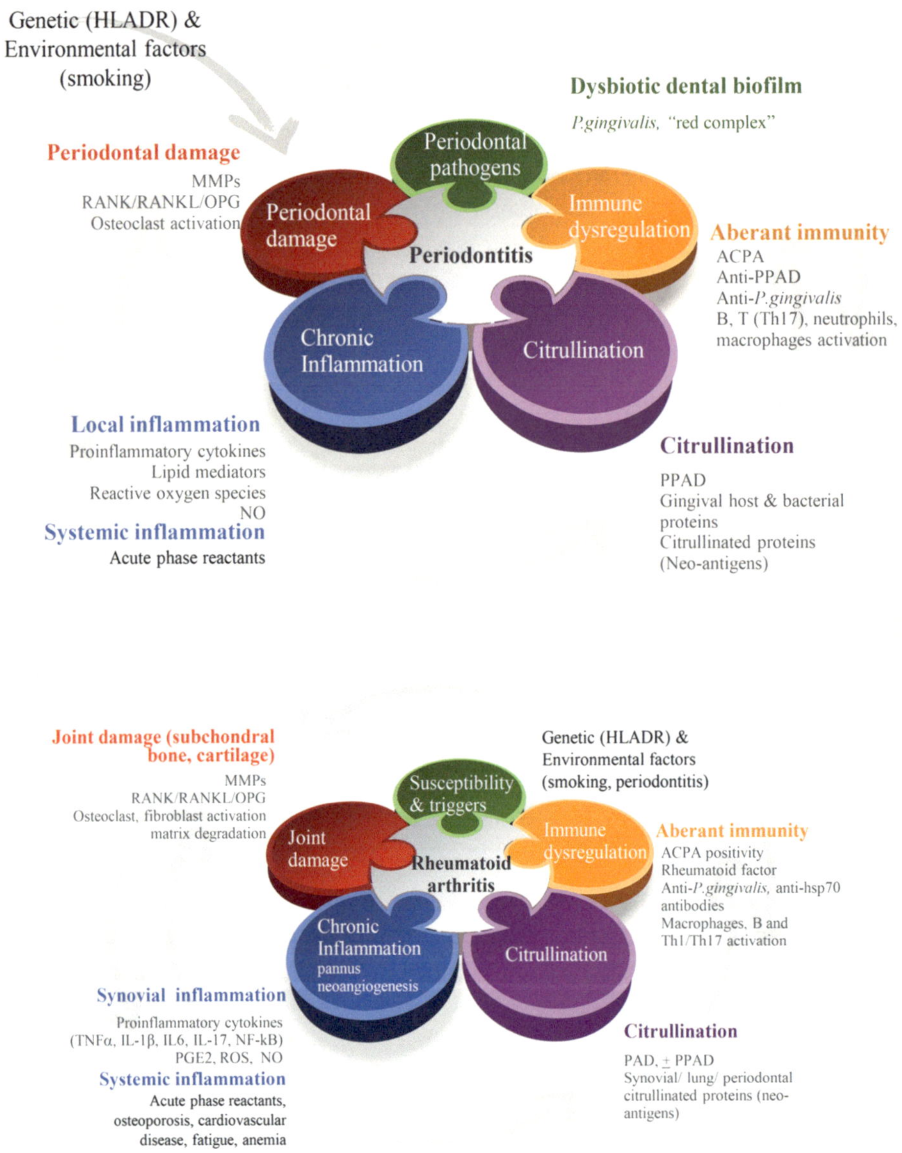

Figure 3. The paradigm of RA—periodontitis pathogenic link.

A 'two-hit' model for the link between periodontitis and systemic diseases including RA have already been proposed by Gloub et al. [4] and recently modified, evoking a sharp cascade of events: induction of severe chronic periodontitis by local and systemic factors in relation to RA ('first hit'), and their mitigation by periodontal host modulating therapy ('second hit') [4].

4.4. Therapeutic interferences in rheumatoid arthritis and chronic periodontitis

Current evidences suggests that periodontal treatment may influence clinical outcomes of RA and vice-versa, stipulating the potential advantage of host-modulating therapy to concomitantly control both disorders [1, 4, 8, 48, 50, 53–57].

4.4.1. Effects of therapy for periodontitis on rheumatoid arthritis disease activity and systemic inflammation

It was advocated that specific therapies for periodontitis not only improve disease activity and severity in RA by removing periodontal infection and gingival inflammation, but also improve patient response to therapeutic drugs [1, 8, 50, 53, 54].

Thus, nonsurgical periodontal therapy was directed to improve both signs and symptoms of active RA as well as periodontal status [1, 8, 12]. Similarly, advanced periodontal treatment with scaling and root planning significantly ameliorated gingival infection and severity of periodontitis, while promoting consistent reduction in acute phase reactants, mainly erythrocyte sedimentation rate, in the RA population [1, 8, 12, 53, 54]. The impact of periodontal treatment on RA seems to be greater in patients with substantial amount of systemic inflammation, particularly if periodontitis intervention therapy combined with adjunctive periodontal host-modulating therapy [4, 12, 53, 54].

Furthermore, a positive influence on RA activity scores, rheumatoid factor and ACPA levels, but also on anti-*P. gingivalis* antibodies was reported following supportive periodontal therapy in patients having concomitant RA and chronic periodontitis [1, 12, 52, 54–56].

The consequences of therapy for periodontal disease on RA status actually reflect on the decrease in systemic inflammation, removal of joint exposure to the infectious trigger and the decline in microbial immune subversion [1, 8, 12].

4.4.2. Effects of conventional therapy for rheumatoid arthritis on periodontal status

On the other hand, different authors concluded that early aggressive RA management with synthetic disease modifying anti-rheumatic drugs (DMARDs) and/or biologic agents aiming to achieve and maintain disease remission according to treat-to-target strategies might also restrict periodontal damage in active periodontitis [1, 8, 12, 54].

It is widely accepted that systematic DMARDs ameliorate periodontal disease burden in RA patients with periodontitis, i.e., they decrease gingival inflammation and periodontal destruction [1, 8, 12, 54]. Moreover, glucocorticoids and TNF antagonists are able to clinically improve periodontal disease in RA patients [1, 8, 12, 54]. Anti-cytokine therapy, specifically anti-TNF agents, may play dual role on synovitis as well as periodontal disease [1, 8, 12, 54, 55], reducing inflammation and mitigating both conditions [1, 4, 8, 12]. However, the role of TNF inhibition on periodontitis outcomes in the absence of periodontal treatment is still controversial [1, 8, 12].

5. Conclusions

There is a significant interplay between periodontitis and rheumatoid arthritis as supported by emerging evidences. Despite common T cell activation, the imbalance between pro-inflammatory and anti-inflammatory cytokine profile, citrullination of endogenous proteins and the resultant bone destruction in specific environments (synovium and gingival tissue), further research is required to assess the exact mechanisms and causative link, as well as to define top therapy.

Author details

Codrina Ancuta[1*], Cristina Iordache[2], Eugen Ancuta[3] and Claudia Mihailov[4]

*Address all correspondence to: codrina_ancuta@yahoo.com

1 2nd Rheumatology Department, Clinical Rehabilitation Hospital, "Grigore T. Popa" University of Medicine and Pharmacy, Iasi, Romania

2 Ergonomics Department, School of Dentistry, "Grigore T. Popa" University of Medicine and Pharmacy, Iasi, Romania

3 Research Department, "Elena Doamna" Clinical Hospital, Iasi, Romania

4 2nd Medical Department, Clinical Port Hospital of Constanta, Faculty of Medicine, 'Ovidius' University of Constanta, Romania

References

[1] Joseph R, Jose Raj MG, Sundareswaran S, et al. Does a biological link exist between periodontitis and rheumatoid arthritis? World J Rheumatology. 2014;4(3):80–87.

[2] Koziel J, Mydel P, Potempa J. The link between periodontal disease and rheumatoid arthritis: an updated review. Curr Rheumatol Rep. 2014;16:408.

[3] Batool H, Afzal N, Shahzad F, Kashif M. Relationship between rheumatoid arthritis and chronic periodontitis. J Med Radiol Pathol Surg. 2016;2:11–14.

[4] Payne JB, Gloub LM, Thiele GM, et al. The link between periodontitis and rheumatoid arthritis: a periodontist's perspective. Curr Oral Health Rep. 2015;2:20–29.

[5] Araujo VM, Melo IM, Lima V. Relationship between periodontitis and rheumatoid arthritis: review of the literature. Mediat Inflam. 2015;259074:1–15.

[6] Fuggle NR, Smith TO, Kaul A, Sofat N. Hand to mouth: a systematic review and metaanalysis of the association between rheumatoid arthritis and periodontitis. Front Immunol. 2016;7(80):1–10.

[7] Saini R. Periodontitis and rheumatoid arthritis: inflammatory relationship. J Pharm Bioallied Sci. 2011;3(3):464–465.

[8] Bingham CO. Round 34: periodontal disease and rheumatoid arthritis [Internet]. 2010 [Updated: 2011]. Available from: http://www.hopkinsarthritis.org/physician-corner/rheumatology-rounds/r. [Accessed: 01-aug-2016]

[9] Detert J, Pischon N, Burmester GR, et al. The association between rheumatoid arthritis and periodontal disease. Arthritis Res Ther. 2010;12:218 (1–7).

[10] Valesini G, Gerardi MC, Iannuccelli C, et al. Citrullination and autoimmunity. Autoimmun Rev. 2015;14(6):490–497.

[11] Hussain M, Stover CM, Dupont A. P. gingivalis in periodontal disease and atherosclerosis—scenes of action for antimicrobial peptides and complement. Front Immunol. 2015;6(45):1–6.

[12] Hein C. A closer look at the association between periodontal disease and rheumatoid arthritis. Dimens Dent Hyg. 2008;6(3):30–33.

[13] van Dyke TE. Commentary: periodontitis is characterized by an immuno-inflamatory host-mediated destruction of bone and connective tissues that support the teeth. J Periodontol. 2014;85:509–511.

[14] Gümüş P, Buduneli E, Başak B, et al. Gingival crevicular fluid, serum levels of receptor PArheumatoid arthritis and osteoporosis and with periodontal disease. J Periodontol. 2013;84(11):1627–1637.

[15] Kobayashi T, Yoshie H. Host responses in the link between periodontitis and rheumatoid arthritis. Curr Oral Health Rep. 2015;2:1–8.

[16] Klareskog L, Malmström V, Lundberg K, et al. Smoking, citrullination and genetic variability in the immunopathogenesis of rheumatoid arthritis. Semin Immunol. 2011;23:92–98.

[17] Catrina AI, Ytterberg AJ, Reynisdottir G, et al. Lungs, joints and immunity against citrullinated proteins in rheumatoid arthritis. Nat Rev Rheumatol. 2014;10:645–653.

[18] Badran Z, Strillou X, Verner C, et al. Periodontitis as a risk factor for systemic disease: are microparticles the missing link? Med Hypotheses. 2015;84(6):555–556.

[19] Mysak J, Podzimek S, Sommerova P, et al. Porphyromonas gingivalis: Major periodontopathic pathogen overview. J Immunol Res.2014;2014:476068.

[20] Maresz KJ, Helvard A, Sroka A, et al. Porphyromonas gingivalis facilitates the development and progression of destructive arthritis through its unique bacterial peptidylarginine deiminase (PAD). PLoS Pathog. 2013;9:81003627.

[21] Hajishengallis G, Liang S, Payne MA, et al. Low-abundance biofilm species orchestrates inflammatory periodontal disease through the commensal microbiota and complement. Cell Host Microbe. 2011;10:497–506.

[22] Leech MT, Bartold PM. The association between rheumatoid arthritis and periodontitis. Best Pract Res Clin Rheumatol. 2015;29:189–201.

[23] Scher JU, Abramson SB. Periodontal disease, Porphyromonas gingivalis, and rheumatoid arthritis: what triggers autoimmunity and clinical disease? Arthritis Res Ther. 2013;15:122(1–3).

[24] Scher JU, Bretz WA, Abramson SB. Periodontal disease and subgingival microbiota as contributors for rheumatoid arthritis pathogenesis: modifiable risck factors? Curr Opin Rheumatol. 2014;26:424–429.

[25] Konig MF, Paracha AS, Moni M, et al. Defining the role of Porphyromonas gingivalis peptidylarginine deiminase (PPAD) in rheumatoid arthritis through the study of PPAD biology. Ann Rheum Dis. 2015;74(11):2054–2061.

[26] Harvey GP, Fitzsmmons TR, Dhamarpatni AA, et al. Expression of peptidylarginine deiminase-2 and-4, citrullinated proteins anti citrullinated protein antibodies in human gingiva. J Periodontal Res. 2013;48:252–261.

[27] Hensvold A-H, Reznisdottir G, Catrina A. From citrullination to specific immunity and disease in rheumatoid arthritis. Protein Deimin Human Health Dis. 2014;2:25–42.

[28] Abdukkah SN, Farmer EA, Spargo L, et al. Porphromonas gingivalis peptidylarginine deiminase substrate specificity. Anaerobe. 2013;23:102–108.

[29] Amara K, Steen J, Murray F, et al. Monoclonal IgG antibodies generated from joint derived B cells of RA patients have a strong bias towards citurllianted autantingen recognition. J Exp Med. 2013;3:445–455.

[30] Quirke AM, Lugli EB, Wegner N, et al. Heightened immune response to autocitrullinated Porphyromonas gingivalis peptidylarginine deiminase: a potential mechanism for breaching immunologic tolerance in rheumatoid arthritis. Ann Rheum Dis. 2014;73(1):263–269.

[31] Andrade F, Darrah E, Gucek M, et al. Autocitrullination of human peptidylarginine deiminase type 4 regulates protein citrullination during cell activation. Arthritis Rheum. 2010;62(6):1630–1640.

[32] Baka Z, György B, Géher P, et al. Citrullination under physiological and pathological conditions. Joint Bone Spine. 2012;79:431–436.

[33] Mikuls TR, Payne JB, Yu F, et al. Periodontitis and porphromonas gingivalis in patients with rheumatoid arthritis. Arthr Rheumatol. 2014;66(5):1090–1100.

[34] Wegner N, Lundberg K, Kinloch A, et al. Autoimmunity to specific citrullinated proteins gives the first clues to the etiology of rheumatoid arthritis. Immunol Rev. 2010;233:34–54.

[35] Arnson Y, Shoenfeld Y, Amita H. Effects of tabacco smoke on immunity, inflammation and autoimmunity. J Autoimmun. 2010;34:258–265.

[36] Lappin DF, Apatzidou D, Quirke AM, et al. Influence of periodontal disease, Porphyromonas gingivalis and cigarette smoking on systemic antic-citrullinated peptide antibody titres. J Clin Periodontol. 2013;40:907–915.

[37] Manivelavan D, Vijayasamundeeswari CK. Anti-cyclic citrullinated peptide antibody: an early diagnostic and prognostic biomarker of rheumatoid arthritis. J Clin Diagn Res. 2012;6(8):1393–1396.

[38] Gottenberg JE, Ravaud P, Cantagrel A, et al. Positivity for anti-cyclic citrullinated peptide is associated with a better response to abatacept: data from the "Orencia and Rheumatoid Arthritis" registry. Ann Rheum Dis. 2012;7(11):1815–1819.

[39] Demoruelle MK, Parish MC, Derber LA, et al. Performance of anti-cyclic citrullinated peptide assazs differs in subjects at increased risk of rheumatoid arthritis and subjects with established disease. Arthritis Rheum. 2013;65:2243–2263.

[40] Gonzales SM, Payne JB, Yu E, et al. Alveolar bone loss is associated with circulating anti-citrullinated proteins antibody (ACPA) in patients with rheumatoid arthritis. J Periodontol. 2015;86(2):221–231.

[41] Ishi PE, Barros Bertolo M, Rossa Jr C, et al. Periodontal condition in patients with rheumatoid arthritis. Braz Oral Res. 2008;22(1):72–77.

[42] Pischon N, Pischon T, Kroger J, et al. Association among rheumatoid arthritis, oral hygiene, and periodontitis. J Periodontol. 2008;79:979–986.

[43] Dissick A, Redman RS, Jones M, et al. Association of periodontitis with rheumatoid arthritis: a pilot study. J Periodontol. 2010;81:223–230.

[44] Joseph R, Rajappan S, Nath SG, et al. Association between chronic periodontitis and rheumatoid arthritis: a hospital-based case-control study. Rheumatol Int. 2013;33(1): 103–109.

[45] Hendler A, Mulli TK, Hughes FJ, et al. Involvement of autoimmunity in the pathogenesis of aggressive periodontitis. J Dent Res. 2010;89:1389–1394.

[46] Seror R, David-Gall S, Bonnaure-Mallet M, et al. Association of anti-Porphromonas gingivalis antibody titers with nonsmoking status in early rheumatoid arthritis: results from the prospective French cohort of patients with early rheumatoid arthritis. Arthr Rheumatol. 2015;67(7):1729–1737.

[47] Kaur S, Bright R, Proudman SM, et al. Does periodontal treatment influence clinical and biochemical measures for rheumatoid arthritis? A systemic review and meta-analysis. Semin Arthr Rheum 2014;44:113–22.

[48] Potikuri D, Dannana KC, Kanchinadam S, et al. Periodontal disease is significantly higher in nonsmoking treatment-naïve rheumatoid arthritis patients: results from a case-control study. Ann Rheum Dis. 2012;71:1541–1544.

[49] Eriksson K, Nise L, Kats A, et al. Prevalence of periodontitis in patients with established rheumatoid arthritis: a Swedish population based case-control study. PLoS One. 2016;11(7):e0155956.

[50] Pinho Mde N, Oliveira RD, Novaes Jr AB, et al. Relationship between periodontitis and rheumatoid arthritis and the effect of non-surgical periodontal treatment. Braz Dent J. 2009;20:355–364.

[51] Bryrkoglu B, Buduneli N, Aksu K, et al. Periodontal therapy in chronic periodontitis lowers gingival crevicular fluid interleukin-1beta and DAS 28 in rheumatoid arthritis patients. Rheumatol Int. 2013;33:2607–2616.

[52] Moutsopoulos NM, Kling HM, Angelov N, et al. Porphromonas gingivalis promotes Th 17 inducing pathways in chronic periodontitis. J Autoimmun. 2012;39:294–303.

[53] Monsarrat P, Vergnes JN, Cantagrel A, et al. Effect of periodontal treatment on the clinical parameters of patients with rheumatoid arthritis: study protocol of the randomized, controlled ESPERA trial. Trials. 2013;14:253(1–9).

[54] Ortis P, Bissada NF, Paloma L, et al. Periodontal therapy reduces the severity of active rheumatoid arthritis in patients treated with or without tumor necrosis factor inhibitors. J Periodontal. 2009;80:535–540.

[55] Okada M, Kobayashi T, Ito S, et al. Periodontal treatment decreases levels of antibodies to porphryromonas gingivalis and citrulline in patients with rheumatoid arthritis and periodontics. J Periodontol. 2013;84(12):e74–e84.

[56] Erciyas K, Sezer U, Ustün K, et al. Effects of periodontal therapy on disease activity and systemic inflammation in rheumatoid arthritis patients. Oral Dis. 2013;19:394–400.

[57] Fisher BA, Cartwright AJ, Quirke AM, et al. Smoking, Porphyromonas gingivalis and the immune response to citrullinated autoantigens before the clinical onset of rheumatoid arthritis in a Southern European nested case-control study. BMC Musculoskelet Disord. 2015;16:331(1–11).

Section 4

Endoplasmic Reticulum and Rheumatoid Arthritis

Chapter 7

Synoviolin is a Novel Pathogenic Factor of Arthropathy and Chronic Inflammation

Naoko Yagishita, Satoko Aratani, Hidetoshi Fujita,
Yoshihisa Yamano, Kusuki Nishioka and
Toshihiro Nakajima

Additional information is available at the end of the chapter

http://dx.doi.org/10.5772/66352

Abstract

Inflammation is classical pathogenic concept, but still very crucial for understanding many disorders even in twenty-first century. The purpose of inflammation is to eliminate the damaged tissues and to initiate tissue repair. By contrast, chronic inflammation leads to intractable diseases, including rheumatoid arthritis (RA), atherosclerosis, cancer, diabetes mellitus, and obesity. We recently cloned synoviolin, an E3 ubiquitin ligase, as an overexpressing molecule in rheumatoid synovium and has been verifying its critical roles in RA, inflammatory cytokine signaling, and fibrosis. Moreover, *synoviolin*-deficient mice exhibited severe anemia caused by defective nursing activity of erythrocytes in the fetal liver. This phenomenon resembles of RA that accelerates nursing activity. Our data indicate a close relationship between embryogenesis and RA. We successfully discovered synoviolin inhibitors, LS-101 and LS-102. These drugs have inhibitory effects to synoviolin in vitro and in vivo. We are now proceeding with the optimization of small compounds, and we hope our research will lead to the development of a new therapy for RA and fibrosis and other synoviolin-related diseases.

Keywords: synoviolin, synoviocyte, ubiquitin ligase, ERAD

1. Introduction

Rheumatoid arthritis (RA) has a tremendous negative impact on quality of life and affects nearly 1% of the adult population worldwide [1, 2].

Clinically, RA is characterized by multiple joint pain, stiffness, and swelling due to synovial inflammation and effusion [3–6]. The pathological features of RA result from multiple processes including chronic inflammation, overgrowth of synovial cells, bone and joint destruction, and as terminal phase tissue fibrosis.

2. Synoviolin is a causative factor for arthropathy

We cloned "synoviolin" by immunoscreening using anti-rheumatoid synovial cell antibody [7]. Synoviolin is a RING-type E3 ubiquitin ligase and is highly expressed in rheumatoid synovial cells [7]. Synoviolin is a mammalian homolog of Hrd1p/Der3p [8–10] and is involved in endoplasmic reticulum(ER)-associated degradation (ERAD) [7].

In eukaryotic cells, the balance of protein synthesis and degradation is strictly regulated, and the selective degradation of protein is carried out *via* the ubiquitin-proteasome system (UPS) [11, 12]. The proteins targeted for proteasomal degradation are ubiquitinated by three enzymes: ubiquitin-activating enzyme E1, ubiquitin-conjugated enzyme E2, and E3 ubiquitin ligases [11, 12]. Newly synthesized proteins are correctly folded in the ER and transported to the secretory pathway. When the amount of misfolded protein exceeds the protein folded capacity, result from ER stresses, it is eliminated by UPS-dependent degradation process of ERAD [13]. Synoviolin plays an important role in ERAD as an E3 ubiquitin ligase and involved in quality control of proteins.

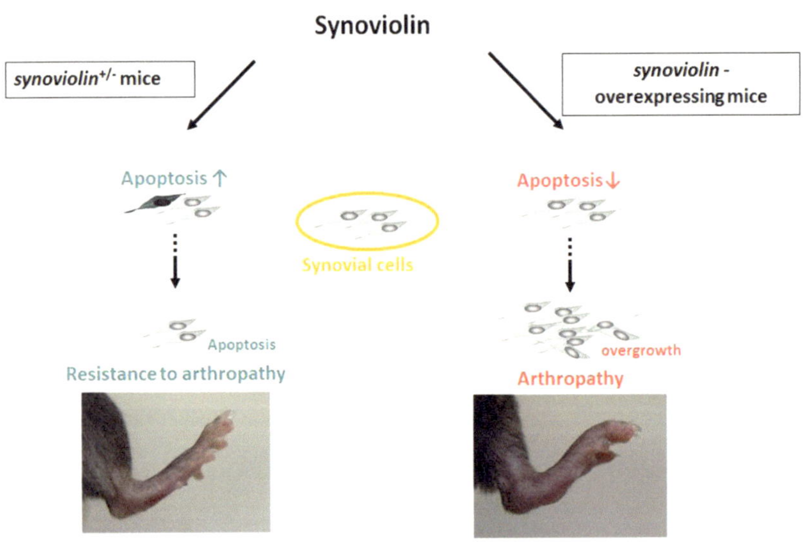

Figure 1. Synoviolin is a causative factor for arthropathy. "Gain-of-function" of synoviolin results in the development of spontaneous arthropathy through the anti-apoptotic effects of synoviolin. On the other hand, *syno*$^{+/-}$ mice are resistant to CIA model. Therefore, synoviolin is a novel causative factor for RA.

http://dx.doi.org/10.5772/66352

Synoviolin is ubiquitously expressed in whole body, especially highly expressed in synoviocytes of patients with RA. Approximately 30% of overexpression of synoviolin in transgenic mice leads to advanced arthropathy caused by reduced apoptosis of synoviocytes (**Figure 1**) [7]. On the other hand, synoviolin-heterozygous mice demonstrate resistance to the development of collagen-induced arthritis (CIA) because of enhanced apoptosis of synovial cells (**Figure 1**) [7]. We postulate that the overexpression of synoviolin leads to hyperactivation of the ERAD and results in synovial hyperplasia. In addition, synoviolin negatively regulates the tumor suppressor p53 in the cytoplasm by ubiquitinating p53 [14]. Therefore, synoviolin regulates both apoptosis in response to ER stress and a p53-dependent apoptotic pathway. These studies indicate that synoviolin is a novel pathogenic factor of arthropathy through its anti-apoptotic effects [15].

3. The reason for death of *syno*$^{-/-}$ mice in utero

To gain insight into the function of synoviolin in vivo, we generated *synoviolin*-deficient (*syno*$^{-/-}$) mice by gene-targeted disruption. Strikingly, all fetuses lacking *synoviolin* died in utero by embryonic day 13.5 (E13.5) [16]. It is surprising that loss of synoviolin only can cause embryonic lethality, since Hrd1p/Del3p, a yeast homolog of synoviolin, is nonessential for survival [8]. Then, why is synoviolin deficiency associated with embryonic death? Morphologically, there was no remarkable difference between E13.5 wild-type and *syno*$^{-/-}$ embryos; however, the *syno*$^{-/-}$ fetal liver looked pale, suggesting an abnormal hematological status in *syno*$^{-/-}$ embryos, since the liver becomes the main hematopoietic organ by E12.5 [17–20]. Indeed, the number of peripheral blood cells was decreased in *syno*$^{-/-}$ embryos, and the level of β-major globin, which first appears in the fetal liver during definitive erythropoiesis, was markedly reduced in *syno*$^{-/-}$ embryos [16]. Subsequently, we examined erythropoiesis in *syno*$^{-/-}$ in vitro by colony-forming assay. Unexpectedly, we found that erythrocyte progenitors of *syno*$^{-/-}$ could differentiate in vitro to produce hemoglobin. Definitive erythropoiesis in embryos is controlled by cell autonomous and non-cell autonomous mechanisms. Therefore, it is expected that the abnormal cell morphology in *syno*$^{-/-}$ erythroid is secondary to changes in the local environment, that is, liver. Consequently, we analyzed the *syno*$^{-/-}$ fetal liver and found reduced number of hepatocytes and their augmented apoptotic cell death in *syno*$^{-/-}$ embryos compared to wild-type embryos [16]. Considered together, the above results indicate that the death in utero of *syno*$^{-/-}$ around E13.5 is caused by abnormal erythropoiesis in a non-cell autonomous manner, which depends on aberrant apoptosis in the liver.

4. Symmetric features of synoviolin in RA and embryogenesis

At a glance, embryogenesis and RA are non-related events. However, when considered through synoviolin, commonness becomes apparent. What is the common feature between these two processes? One answer could be the nurse-like cells. Nurse cells were first recognized in a cell suspension from the thymus [21, 22]. Wekere and Ketelsen concluded that thymic nurse cells played an important role in the differentiation of thymocytes [23–25]. They referred to this phenomenon as pseudoemperipolesis. Pseudoemperipolesis has been observed also in the interaction between murine lymphocytes and murine bone marrow (BM) stromal cells [23–25]. Iwagami et al. [26] and Shimaoka et al. [27] reported cloning of nurse cells from synovial tissue of patients with RA. Moreover, BM stromal cells migrated from the BM into the affected joint cavity and contribute to synovial proliferation [28]. Clinically, BM stromal cells derived from donors show very little pseudoemperipoletic activity, and thus, nurse cell activity is considered a unique feature of BM stromal cells derived from RA [29]. That is, RA is a disease with accelerated nurse cell activity of BM stromal cells. In other words, increased nursing cell activity would enhance the cooperation between surrounding cells, BM stromal cells, and synovial cells.

When one compares RA with *syno*$^{-/-}$, these processes are symmetrical. In *syno*$^{-/-}$ fetal liver, there is a complete loss of nurse activity to erythrocytes. The excessive amount of synoviolin in RA and the lack of synoviolin in *syno*$^{-/-}$ are quite a symmetrical feature. These observations suggest the possible involvement of synoviolin in promoting the nursing activity in RA, a topic for future research. A more thorough analysis of *syno*$^{-/-}$ indicates that RA and embryogenesis are closely related processes (**Figure 2**).

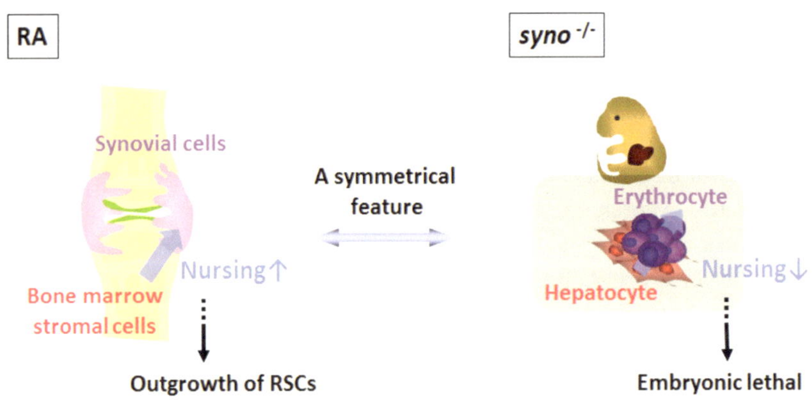

Figure 2. RA and embryogenesis have shared features. RA is a disease with accelerated nursing activity of bone marrow stromal cells. On the other hand, *syno*$^{-/-}$ fetal liver shows loss of nursing cell activity of erythrocytes. In this regard, RA and *syno*$^{-/-}$ demonstrate a symmetrical feature. The study of *syno*$^{-/-}$ has allowed the elucidation of new etiological factors of RA.

5. Impact of synoviolin on RA and embryogenesis

Embryogenesis, in which a single fertilized egg forms an individual consisting of millions of cells, is the most complicated process in higher eukaryote. That synoviolin shoulders this process highlights the importance of this protein. On the other hand, RA is a complex disease, in which all the details of its pathology are not yet understood. That this fundamental molecule is involved in the crisis of RA makes it conceivable that synoviolin is implicated in the intricacy of this disease. Furthermore, the joint cavity, representing the nidus of RA, is a complex space; it is formed of several types of cells, such as synovial cells, chondrocytes, osteoblasts, osteoclasts, and bone marrow cells. Just as there are many contacts with all sorts of cells in embryogenesis, the same is true for contacts between these numerous types of cells in the RA joint cavity. Except for the joint and eye, there is no space in our body formed by so many types of cells. In this regard, RA is a disorder of this complex space which needs to connect with the periphery, and the crisis of RA requires making sense of synoviolin function. Therefore, analysis of $syno^{-/-}$ has indicated that synoviolin is a molecule that connects embryogenesis and RA, and studies involving both processes would be the cutting edge in elucidating the pathogenesis of RA.

6. Synoviolin is participated in multiple processes of RA

RA consists of multiple processes including chronic inflammation, overgrowth of synovial cells, bone and joint destruction, and tissue fibrosis. Synoviolin plays an important role in over growth of synovial cells through hyperactivation of ERAD.

Inflammation is the most important process of RA. The synovial cells, macrophages, T cells, and B cells produce many kinds of cytokines, such as interleukin (IL)-1, IL-6, IL-10, tumor necrosis factor (TNF), and transforming growth factor β (TGF-β), and these cytokines stimulate the overgrowth of synovial cells [3–6]. Because it forms pannus, a mass of synovial tissue, inflammation leads to destruction of the bone and cartilage [3–6].

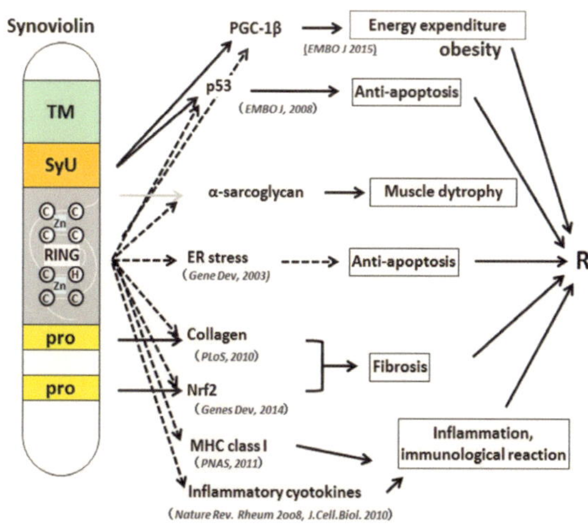

Figure 3. Synoviolin and its related disorders. The scientific summary of synoviolin function. Synoviolin is involved in a lot of disorders and would be a potential candidate for new drug of these disorders. Our compounds which inhibit the activity of synoviolin would be useful for these disorders. TM: transmembrane domain; SyU: SyU domain (amino acids, aa 236–270 of synoviolin); pro: prolin-rich region.

With regard to the relationship between synoviolin and inflammation, it was reported that IL-17 induction of synoviolin may contribute to RA chronicity [30], and synoviolin targets misfolded MHC class I heavy chains [31] and is a positive regulator of T-cell immunity [32]. Toh et al. demonstrated that synoviolin levels are elevated in circulating monocytes of RA patients [33]. It was reported that dual blockade of TNF and IL-17 decreased disease progression more effectively than when only one cytokine was blocked [34]. Therefore, it was suggested that synoviolin would be a potential candidate for new drug of chronic inflammation (**Figure 3**).

7. Synoviolin is also involved in fibrosis

Fibrosis is the terminal pathological feature of RA and results from excessive accumulation of the extracellular matrix (ECM) such as collagen and fibronectin [35]. Fibrosis is also major a pathological feature of chronic inflammatory disease. We previously demonstrated that synoviolin is upregulated in hepatic stellate cells (HSCs) of human cirrhosis, and synoviolin-heterozygous mice are resistant to CCl_4-induced hepatic injury [36]. Moreover, procollagen was abnormally accumulated in the ER of synoviolin-deficient mouse embryonic fibroblasts, suggesting the involvement of synoviolin in collagen secretion [36]. We also demonstrated that synoviolin expression and collagen secretion are enhanced in lung fibrosis using in vitro model, in which A549 human lung adenocarcinoma cells were transfected with exon-4 deleted surfactant protein C [37], which has been reported to induce ER stress [38, 39]. Li et al. demonstrated that synoviolin is involved in the renal fibrosis using the unilateral ureteral obstruction (UUO) model and plays an important role in the maturation of collagen [40]. These reports indicated that synoviolin plays an important role in fibrosis through the collagen expression and secretion (**Figure 3**).

8. Synoviolin as a therapeutic target for RA

During the past decade, biological agents have been approved for clinical use and dramatically have changed the treatment of RA. However, in some cases, patients fail to respond to the biologic treatment. It was reported that synoviolin overexpression of RA patients was associated with nonresponse to infliximab treatment (a monoclonal antibody against TNFα) [33]. Moreover, these agents are associated with high costs and discomfort arising from subcutaneous or intravenous administration. Thus, there is a clear need for the development of cheaper, orally administrated therapies with fewer side effects.

Since synoviolin is a pathogenic factor for chronic inflammation including RA and fibrosis (**Figure 3**), inhibition of synoviolin activity may be a useful therapeutic approach for the treatment of RA. Then, synoviolin is a drug-able molecule because: (1) synoviolin is an enzyme; (2) synoviolin localizes in cytoplasm; (3) the structure of synoviolin has been determined

(Nakajima T, unpublished data); and (4) specific substrates of synoviolin have been identified such as p53 [14]. Moreover, synoviolin may be a disease-modifying molecule because synoviolin may be involved in RA and fibrosis and may be implicated in some severe diseases such as interstitial pneumonia and systemic sclerosis. In making synoviolin a therapeutic target, downregulation of synoviolin and/or inhibition of its activity might be useful.

In order to reduce the amount of synoviolin, it is important to elucidate the transcriptional regulation of synoviolin. Establishing the mechanisms of transcriptional regulation of synoviolin should allow suppression of synoviolin transcription. We identified Ets binding site in the *synoviolin* proximal promoter as for crucial site of synoviolin expression. Moreover, the GA-binding protein (GABP) α/β complex is essential for its transcriptional regulation [41].

9. Development of synoviolin inhibitors

Next, in order to block the enzymatic activity of synoviolin, we performed high-throughput screening that inhibits the auto-ubiquitination activity of synoviolin. Over four million compounds from Pharmacopeia's compound collection were screened, and we found two unique compounds, termed LS-101 and LS-102 [42]. LS-101 and LS-102 demonstrated an inhibition of synoviolin auto-ubiquitination with IC_{50} of ~15 and 20 μM, respectively. LS-101 demonstrates stronger efficacy than LS-102, but less selectivity to synoviolin among other RING-type E3 ubiquitin ligases. Administration of either LS-101 or LS-102 also suppressed the clinical severity scores in mice collagen-induced arthritis (CIA) model. There was no difference in the protective effect between high dose of LS-101 and LS-102.

Moreover, it was also reported that LS-102 was able to suppress CCl_4-induced elevation of alanine aminotransferase (ALT) and restored normal liver morphology in CCl_4-induced liver cirrhosis mice model [43]. We also demonstrated that collagen secretion is suppressed by LS-102 in lung fibrosis using in vitro model [37]. Therefore, LS-102 is a novel potential drug for synoviolin inhibition. Thus, we proceed toward the optimization of LS-101 and LS-102 and get the derivative compounds from these compounds named LS-302 (Nakajima T, unpublished data). The arthritis scores of mice injected with LS-302 were also decreased. We hope our research will lead to the development of a new therapy for synoviolin-related diseases and serve as an example for the therapeutic benefit from E3 ligase inhibitors.

According to the UPS, a proteasome inhibitor has been developed. Bortezomib (BTZ) is the first proteasome inhibitor to gain the U.S. Food and Drug Administration (FDA) approval [44, 45]. BTZ induces apoptosis of a wide variety of cancer cells, and however, there are some patients who do not respond to therapy [44, 46]. There are second-generation proteasome inhibitors: carfilzomib [44, 47–49], ixazomib [44, 47, 48, 50], delanzomib [44, 47, 48, 51], oprozomib [44, 47, 48, 52], and marizomib [44, 48, 53]. These drugs are global inhibitors of the proteasome, and therefore, the associated toxicities prevent their use for the treatment of chronic disease such as RA. It is important to develop inhibitors of the UPS enzymatic cascade, and E3 ubiquitin ligase is suitable target given their large number and substrate specificity [54].

There is HDM2, the E3 ubiquitin ligase that regulates the degradation of p53 [55, 56], inhibitor currently in clinical trials [57, 58]. Then, synoviolin inhibitor would be a drug that follows a HDM.

Acknowledgements

This work was supported by JSPS KAKENHI Grant Number 20689019, 23659502, 26461478, 20249052, 20059033, 20013045, by grant from Takeda Science Foundation.

Author details

Naoko Yagishita[1], Satoko Aratani[2,3,4], Hidetoshi Fujita[2,3], Yoshihisa Yamano[1], Kusuki Nishioka[2] and Toshihiro Nakajima[1,2,3,4,5,6*]

*Address all correspondence to: marlin@tokyo-med.ac.jp

1 Department of Rare Diseases Research, Institute of Medical Science, St. Marianna University School of Medicine, Kawasaki, Kanagawa, Japan

2 Institute of Medical Science, Tokyo Medical University, Shinjuku-ku, Tokyo, Japan

3 Department of Future Medical Science, Institute of Medical Science, Tokyo Medical University, Shinjuku-ku, Tokyo, Japan

4 Physician, Student and Researcher Support Center, Tokyo Medical University, Shinjuku-ku, Tokyo, Japan

5 Integrated Genome Editing Section (iGES), Tokyo Medical University, Shinjuku-ku, Tokyo, Japan

6 Bayside Misato Medical Center, Niida, Kochi, Japan

References

[1] Harris ED. Rheumatoid arthritis. Pathophysiology and implications for therapy. N Engl J Med 1990; 322: 1277–1289.

[2] Feldmann M, Brennan FM, Maini RN. Rheumatoid arthritis. Cell 1996; 85: 307–310.

[3] Stanczyk J, Ospelt C, Gay RE, Gay S. Synovial cell activation. Curr Opin Rheumatol 2006; 18: 262–267.

http://dx.doi.org/10.5772/66352

[4] McInnes IB, Schett G. Cytokines in the pathogenesis of rheumatoid arthritis. Nat Rev Immunol 2007; 7: 429–442.

[5] McInnes IB, Schett G. The pathogenesis of rheumatoid arthritis. N Engl J Med 2011; 365: 2205–2219.

[6] Furst DE, Emery P. Rheumatoid arthritis pathophysiology: update on emerging cytokine and cytokine-associated cell targets. Rheumatology 2014; 53: 1560–1569.

[7] Amano T, Yamasaki S, Yagishita N, Tsuchimochi K, Shin H, Kawahara K, Aratani S, Fujita H, Zhang L, Ikeda R, Fujii R, Miura N, Komiya S, Nishioka K, Maruyama I, Fukamizu A, Nakajima T. Synoviolin/Hrd1, an E3 ubiquitin ligase, as a novel pathogenic factor for arthropathy. Genes Dev 2003; 17: 2436–2449.

[8] Bordallo J, Plemper RK, Finger A, Wolf DH. Der3p/Hrd1p is required for endoplasmic reticulum-associated degradation of misfolded lumenal and integral membrane proteins. Mol Biol Cell 1998; 9: 209–222.

[9] Shearer AG. Hampton, RY. Structural control of endoplasmic reticulum-associated degradation: effect of chemical chaperones on 3-hydroxy-3-methylglutaryl-CoA reductase. J Biol Chem 2004; 279: 188–196.

[10] Shearer AG. Hampton RY. Lipid-mediated, reversible misfolding of a sterol-sensing domain protein. EMBO J 2005; 24: 149–159.

[11] Hershko A, Ciechanover A. The ubiquitin system. Annu Rev Biochem 1998; 67: 425–479.

[12] Pickart CM. Mechanisms underlying ubiquitination. Annu Rev Biochem 2001; 70: 503–533.

[13] Morito D, Nagata K. Pathogenic hijacking of ER-associated degradation: is ERAD flexible? Mol Cell 2015; 59: 335–344.

[14] Yamasaki S, Yagishita N, Sasaki T, Nakazawa M, Kato Y, Yamadera T, Bae E, Toriyama S, Ikeda R, Zhang L, Fujitani K, Yoo E, Tsuchimochi K, Ohta T, Araya N, Fujita H, Aratani S, Eguchi K, Komiya S, Maruyama I, Higashi N, Sato M, Senoo H, Ochi T, Yokoyama S, Amano T, Kim J, Gay S, Fukamizu A, Nishioka K, Tanaka K, Nakajima T. Cytoplasmic destruction of p53 by the endoplasmic reticulum-resident ubiquitin ligase 'Synoviolin'. EMBO J 2007; 26: 113–122.

[15] Yagishita N, Yamasaki S, Nishioka K, Nakajima T. Synoviolin, protein folding and the maintenance of joint homeostasis. Nat Clin Pract Rheumatol 2008; 4: 91–97.

[16] Yagishita N, Ohneda K, Amano T, Yamasaki S, Sugiura A, Tsuchimochi K, Shin H, Kawahara K, Ohneda O, Ohta T, Tanaka S, Yamamoto M, Maruyama I, Nishioka K, Fukamizu A, Nakajima T. Essential Role of Synoviolin in Embryogenesis. J Biol Chem 2005; 280: 7909–7916.

[17] Ito E, Toki T, Ishihara H, Ohtani H, Gu L, Yokoyama M, Engel JD, Yamamoto M. Erythroid transcription factor GATA-1 is abundantly transcribed in mouse testis. Nature 1993; 362: 466–468.

[18] Ohneda K, Yamamoto M. Roles of hematopoietic transcription factors GATA-1 and GATA-2 in the development of red blood cell lineage. Acta Haematol 2002; 108: 237–45.

[19] Shimizu R, Takahashi S, Ohneda K, Engel JD, Yamamoto M. In vivo requirements for GATA-1 functional domains during primitive and definitive erythropoiesis. EMBO J 2001; 20: 5250–5261.

[20] Zon LI. Developmental biology of hematopoiesis. Blood 1995; 86: 2876–2891.

[21] Wekerle H, Ketelsen UP. Thymic nurse cells: Ia-bearing epithelium involved in T-lymphocyte differentiation? Nature 1980; 283: 402–404.

[22] Wekerle H, Ketelsen UP, Ernst M. Thymic nurse cells. Lymphoepithelial cell complexes in murine thymus: morphological and serological characterization. J Exp Med 1980; 151: 925–944.

[23] Witte PL, Robinson M, Henley A, Low MG, Stiers DL, Perkins S, Fleischman RA, Kincade PW. Relationships between B-lineage lymphocytes and stromal cells in long-term bone marrow cultures. Eur J Immunol 1987; 17: 1473–1484.

[24] Miyake K, Hasunuma Y, Yagita H, Kimoto M. Requirement for VLA-4 and VLA-5 integrins in lymphoma cells binding to and migration beneath stromal cells in culture. J Cell Biol 1992; 119: 653–662.

[25] Makrynikola V, Bianchi A, Bradstock K, Gottlieb D, Hewson J. Migration of acute lymphoblastic leukemia cells into human bone marrow stroma. Leukemia 1994; 8: 1734–1743.

[26] Iwagami S, Furue S, Toyosaki T, Horikawa T, Doi H, Satomi S, Itoh T, Sakata T, Suzuki R. Establishment and characterization of nurse cell-like clones from human skin. Nurse cell-like clones can stimulate autologous mixed lymphocyte reaction. J Immunol 1994; 153: 2927–2938.

[27] Shimaoka Y, Attrep JF, Hirano T, Ishihara K, Suzuki R, Toyosaki T, Ochi T, Lipsky PE. Nurse-like cells from bone marrow and synovium of patients with rheumatoid arthritis promote survival and enhance function of human B cells. J Clin Invest 1998; 102: 606–618.

[28] Nakagawa S, Toritsuka Y, Wakitani S, Denno K, Tomita T, Owaki H, Kimura T, Shino K, Ochi T. Bone marrow stromal cells contribute to synovial cell proliferation in rats with collagen induced arthritis. J Rheumatol 1996; 23: 2098–2103.

[29] Tomita T, Takeuchi E, Toyosaki-Maeda T, Oku H, Kaneko M, Takano H, Sugamoto K, Ohzono K, Suzuki R, Ochi T. Establishment of nurse-like stromal cells from bone marrow of patients with rheumatoid arthritis: indication of characteristic bone marrow

microenvironment in patients with rheumatoid arthritis. Rheumatology 1999; 38: 854–863.

[30] Toh ML, Gonzales G, Koenders MI, Tournadre A, Boyle D, Lubberts E, Zhou Y, Firestein GS, van den Berg WB, Miossec P. Role of interleukin 17 in arthritis chronicity through survival of synoviocytes via regulation of synoviolin expression. PLoS One 2010; 5: e13416.

[31] Burr ML, van den Boomen DJ, Bye H, Antrobus R, Wiertz EJ, Lehner PJ. MHC class I molecules are preferentially ubiquitinated on endoplasmic reticulum luminal residues during HRD1 ubiquitin E3 ligase-mediated dislocation. Proc Natl Acad Sci U S A. 2013; 110: 14290–14295.

[32] Xu Y, Zhao F, Qiu Q, Chen K, Wei J, Kong Q, Gao B, Melo-Cardenas J, Zhang B, Zhang J, Song J, Zhang DD, Zhang J, Fan Y, Li H, Fang D. The ER membrane-anchored ubiquitin ligase Hrd1 is a positive regulator of T-cell immunity. Nat Commun 2016; 15: 1–13.

[33] Toh ML, Marotte H, Blond JL, Jhumka U, Eljaafari A, Mougin B, Miossec, P. Overexpression of synoviolin in peripheral blood and synoviocytes from rheumatoid arthritis patients and continued elevation in nonresponders to infliximab treatment. Arthritis Rheum 2006; 54: 2109–2118.

[34] Koenders MI, Marijnissen RJ, Devesa I, Lubberts E, Joosten LA, Roth J, van Lent PL, van de Loo FA, van den Berg WB. Tumor necrosis factor-interleukin-17 interplay induces S100A8, interleukin-1β, and matrix metalloproteinases, and drives irreversible cartilage destruction in murine arthritis: rationale for combination treatment during arthritis. Arthritis Rheum 2011; 63: 2329–2339.

[35] Wynn TA, Ramalingam TR. Mechanisms of fibrosis: therapeutic translation for fibrotic disease. Nat Med 2012; 18: 1028–1240.

[36] Hasegawa D, Fujii R, Yagishita N, Matsumoto N, Aratani S, Izumi T, Azakami K, Nakazawa M, Fujita H, Sato T, Araya N, Koike J, Tadokoro M, Suzuki N, Nagata K, Senoo H, Friedman SL, Nishioka K, Yamano Y, Itoh F, Nakajima T. E3 ubiquitin ligase synoviolin is involved in liver fibrogenesis. PLoS One 2010; 5: e13590.

[37] Nakajima F, Aratani S, Fujita H, Yagishita N, Ichinose S, Makita K, Setoguchi Y, Nakajima T. Synoviolin inhibitor LS-102 reduces endoplasmic reticulum stress-induced collagen secretion in an in vitro model of stress-related interstitial pneumonia. Int J Mol Med 2015; 35: 110–116.

[38] Nogee LM. Genetics of the hydrophobic surfactant proteins. Biochim Biophys Acta 1998; 1408: 323–333.

[39] Mulugeta S, Nguyen V, Russo SJ, Muniswamy M, Beers MF. A surfactant protein C precursor protein BRICHOS domain mutation causes endoplasmic reticulum stress,

proteasome dysfunction, and caspase 3 activation. Am J Respir Cell Mol Biol 2005; 32: 521–530.

[40] Li L, Shen Y, Ding Y, Liu Y, Su D, Liang X. Hrd1 participates in the regulation of collagen I synthesis in renal fibrosis. Mol Cell Biochem 2014; 386: 35–44.

[41] Tsuchimochi K, Yagishita N, Yamasaki S, Amano T, Kato Y, Kawahara K, Aratani S, Fujita H, Ji F, Sugiura A, Izumi T, Sugamiya A, Maruyama I, Fukamizu A, Komiya S, Nishioka K, Nakajima T. Identification of a crucial site for synoviolin expression. Mol Cell Biol 2005; 25: 7344–7356.

[42] Yagishita N, Aratani S, Leach C, Amano T, Yamano Y, Nakatani K, Nishioka K, Nakajima T. RING-finger type E3 ubiquitin ligase inhibitors as novel candidates for the treatment of rheumatoid arthritis. Int J Mol Med 2012; 30: 1281–1286.

[43] Wu T, Zhao F, Gao B, Tan C, Yagishita N, Nakajima T, Wong PK, Chapman E, Fang D, Zhang DD. Hrd1 suppresses Nrf2-mediated cellular protection during liver cirrhosis. Genes Dev 2014; 28: 708–722.

[44] Dou QP, Zonder JA. Overview of proteasome inhibitor-based anti-cancer therapies: perspective on bortezomib and second generation proteasome inhibitors versus future generation inhibitors of ubiquitin-proteasome system. Curr Cancer Drug Targets 2014; 14: 517–536.

[45] Hou YC, Deng JY. Role of E3 ubiquitin ligases in gastric cancer. World J Gastroenterol 2015; 21: 786–793.

[46] Lü S, Wang J. The resistance mechanisms of proteasome inhibitor bortezomib. Biomark Res 2013; 1: 13

[47] Teicher BA, Tomaszewski JE. Proteasome inhibitors. Biochem Pharmacol 2015; 96: 1–9.

[48] Allegra A, Alonci A, Gerace D, Russo S, Innao V, Calabrò L, Musolino C. New orally active proteasome inhibitors in multiple myeloma. Leuk Res 2014; 38: 1–9.

[49] McBride A, Klaus JO, Stockerl-Goldstein K. Carfilzomib: a second-generation proteasome inhibitor for the treatment of multiple myeloma. Am J Health Syst Pharm 2015; 72: 353–360.

[50] Gentile M, Offidani M, Vigna E, Corvatta L, Recchia AG, Morabito L, Morabito F, Gentili S. Ixazomib for the treatment of multiple myeloma. Expert Opin Investig Drugs 2015; 24: 1287–1298.

[51] Berkers CR, Leestemaker Y, Schuurman KG, Ruggeri B, Jones-Bolin S, Williams M, Ovaa H. Probing the specificity and activity profiles of the proteasome inhibitors bortezomib and delanzomib. Mol Pharm 2012; 9: 1126–1135.

[52] Semren N, Habel-Ungewitter NC, Fernandez IE, Königshoff M, Eickelberg O, Stöger T, Meiners S. Validation of the 2nd generation proteasome inhibitor oprozomib for local therapy of pulmonary fibrosis. PLoS One 2015; 10: e0136188.

[53] Ma L, Diao A. Marizomib, a potent second generation proteasome inhibitor from natural origin. Anticancer Agents Med Chem 2015; 15: 298–306.

[54] Deshaies RJ, Joazeiro CA. RING domain E3 ubiquitin ligases. Annu Rev Biochem 2009; 78: 399–434.

[55] Haupt Y, Maya R, Kazaz A, Oren M. Mdm2 promotes the rapid degradation of p53. Nature 1997; 387: 296–299.

[56] Brooks CL, Gu W. p53 ubiquitination: Mdm2 and beyond. Mol Cell 2006; 21: 307–315.

[57] Issaeva N, Bozko P, Enge M, Protopopova M, Verhoef LG, Masucci M, Pramanik A, Selivanova G. Small molecule RITA binds to p53, blocks p53-HDM-2 interaction and activates p53 function in tumors. Nature Medicine 2004; 10: 1321–1328.

[58] Goldenberg SJ, Marblestone JG, Mattern MR, Nicholson B. Strategies for the identification of ubiquitin ligase inhibitors. Biochem Soc Trans 2010; 38: 132–136.

Section 5

Factors as Biomarkers in Rheumatoid Arthritis

Chapter 8

YKL-40: The Search for New Biomarkers in Rheumatoid Arthritis

Maria H. Kazakova and Victoria S. Sarafian

Additional information is available at the end of the chapter

http://dx.doi.org/10.5772/66832

Abstract

There is a need for biomarkers to detect early joint inflammation and destruction of cartilage in different types of arthritis. YKL-40, a 39 kDa heparin- and chitin-binding secreted glycoprotein (also known as human cartilage gp39), has been recently discovered. Its exact biological function is still unclear. Specific receptors for YKL-40 have not been identified yet. The clinical significance of YKL-40 as a biomarker is discussed in different aspects. High level of YKL-40 is found in various human i`nflammatory and neoplastic diseases. We present a review highlighting the information available on YKL-40 and its significance in inflammatory joint diseases, like rheumatoid arthritis (RA). We also report original personal data on the topic concerning YKL-40 levels in serum and synovial fluid of patients with RA in comparison with ultrasonographic parameters and cytokine levels. The findings suggest that YKL-40 might be implicated in the pathogenesis of the disease and could indicate the level of joint inflammation.

Keywords: YKL-40, biomarkers, ultrasonography, cytokines, chitinases

1. Introduction

Identification of new biomarkers would be beneficial for improving biomedical research and drug development. Understanding the relationship between biological processes and clinical outcomes is significant for choosing optimal therapy [1].

A "biomarker" is "a characteristic that is objectively measured and evaluated as an indicator of normal biological processes, pathogenic processes, or pharmacological responses to a therapeutic intervention" [2]. The acceptance of novel biomarkers in clinical settings requires detailed validation process before they could be used in routine clinical practice.

Utility of new biomarkers depends on several aspects: whether the method for detection of the biomarker is a specific, sensitive, fast, and affordable, if the level of the biomarker provides new information about the disease, if the concentration of the biomarker could help the patient's treatment [3].

The current review summarizes our investigations and presents evidences for the role of YKL-40 in the diagnosis and prognosis monitoring of rheumatoid arthritis (RA).

2. YKL-40: gene, protein, regulation, and proposed functions

2.1. YKL-40: protein and gene

YKL-40 is a glycoprotein that is encoded by the *CHI3L1* gene and belongs to the mammalian chitinase-like proteins [4].

Chitinases are enzymes that digest chitin, providing cellular and tissue remodeling during homeostasis in fungi, helminths, insects, and crustaceans [5]. Mammals express both enzymatically active chitinases and enzymatically inactive chitinase-like proteins. The exact biologic role of chitinase-like proteins, such as human YKL-40 protein, is still unclear.

YKL-40 was found out in 1989 as the most abundant protein secreted by MG63 human osteosarcoma cell line [6]. It is also known as human cartilage glycoprotein-39 [4], chitinase 3-like-1 protein [7], chondrex [8], and breast regression protein 39 kDa [9].

The human *YKL-40* gene is located on chromosome 1q32.1 and consists of 10 exons [7]. The promoter sequence contains binding sites for several known factors. The Sp1-family transcription factor had a dominant role in controlling YKL-40 promoter activity [10]. It contains a single polypeptide chain, comprising 383 amino acids, where the three N-terminal amino acids are Y (tyrosine), K (lysine), and L (leucine) and had a molecular mass of 40 kDa [4]. Two mutations of the catalytic glutamic and aspartic acids to leucine and to alanine, respectively, are responsible for the lack of hydrolase activity of YKL-40 [10]. The crystallographic structure of human YKL-40 exhibits two globular domains, forming a groove which corresponds to the active cite of the protein [10].

2.2. YKL-40 ligands

Recent studies suggested different ligands for YKL-40. It was determined that the glycoprotein could facilitate the cross-link between syndecan-1 and integrin [11]. Syndecan-1 is a heparan sulfate proteoglycan acting as a transmembrane receptor. Its coupling with other receptors such as integrins might induce cell adhesion and angiogenesis [12]. It was suggested that YKL-40 could activate key signaling cascades—PI3K/AKT and MAPK/ERK resulting in high rate of cell proliferation and tumor cell survival [13, 14].

These signaling pathways could promote proliferation of synoviocytes and altered innate immunity in inflammatory arthritis [15, 16]. Kjaergaard et al. [17] suggested that another heparan sulfate proteoglycan, perlecan, might be a possible ligand for YKL-40. It was revealed that perlecan comprised distinct effects on angiogenesis dependent on integrin coupling [17, 18].

It was shown that lectin-glycan associations determined the organization of plasma membrane and modulated interactions between surface glycoproteins and receptors [19]. Recently, He et al. [20] identified the interleukin-13 subunit $\alpha2$ (IL-13Raα2) as a possible receptor for YKL-40. They found that the activation of YKL-40 was not dependent on interaction with IL-13Raα2, suggesting that a coreceptor should be considered. The authors supposed that IL-13, IL-13Raα2, and Chi3l1/YKL-40/formed a multimeric complex, but they did not provide details [20].

Still unanswered questions are as follows: how YKL-40 interacts with perlecan? how IL-13, YKL-40, and IL-13Rα2 cooperate? whether the glycoprotein binds to other receptors?

2.3. YKL-40 regulation

Studies focused on YKL-40 regulation revealed controversial data and diverse effects.

Insulin growth factor-I (IGF-I) and insulin growth factor-II (IGF-II) were shown to trigger YKL-40 secretion in guinea pig chondrocytes but not in human chondrocytes [21, 22]. The results might be due to differences in the investigated species.

Proinflammatory interleukins, such as IL-2, IL-6, IL-12, IL-13, IL-17, and IL-18, did not induce YKL-40 transcription in astrocytes [23], while IL-6 and IL-17 showed enhanced production in human primary chondrocyte culture [22, 24].

Different kinds of stressors (hypoxia, ionizating radiation, treatment with TNF-α, bFGF, p53 inhibition, serum depletion) were shown to influence YKL-40 induction on three human malignant glioma cell lines:U87, U118, and U373 [25]. It was found that corticosteroids inhibited YKL-40 protein and mRNA levels in subsets of macrophages (proinflammatory or classically activated macrophages) [26]. Zhang et al. determined that resveratrol inhibited YKL-40 expression by influencing its promoter activity and mRNA transcription levels in U87 cells in vitro [27].

Alterations in the extracellular microenvironment also alter YKL-40 synthesis. Microarray gene expression analysis showed that the gene was overexpressed in dedifferentiated human fetal chondrocytes in comparison with differentiated chondrocytes [28].

YKL-40 secretion is activated by cartilage resection or by replacement of chondrocytes from their native environment. The level of YKL-40 secreted by normal cartilage explants is low during the first day of culture and increases significantly after a few days [22].

A study on the expression of YKL-40 in normal mouse mammary gland development found that YKL-40 was upregulated in ductal epithelial cells. The glycoprotein had the ability to inhibit epithelial secretion and differentiation and to facilitate cell migration under hormone stimulation [29].

The available data regarding the regulation of YKL-40 are quite controversial. These results emphasize the differences in *in vitro* and *in vivo* effects of YKL-40 on cellular and systemic response. We could suggest that YKL-40 might play various roles depending on the cell type it is expressed by.

2.4. Proposed functions for YKL-40

Little is known about the functions of YKL-40 in normal conditions. The glycoprotein is detected during early human embryonic development which is related to rapid proliferation and morphogenetic changes [30].

There is no fixed reference value for YKL-40 in healthy people. It was determined that the level of the glycoprotein increased with age, and it was assumed to be used with an age-matched control group [31]. Johansen proposed serum YKL-40 concentration higher than 20% to be considered as elevated [32]. Published levels of YKL-40 in healthy individuals differ among populations [33–35] and are shown in **Table 1**. We could speculate that divergent YKL-40 levels could be explained with differences in sample collection and assays, genetic polymorphisms, or even epigenetics.

Researchers suggest that YKL-40 protects the extracellular matrix during tissue remodeling via suppression of different types of metalloproteinases [40]. Another study showed that the glycoprotein defined which cells to survive during mammary involution [41] and provided protection against apoptosis [42].

YKL-40 was supposed to induce signaling cascades in connective tissue and functioned as a growth factor for synovial cells and chondrocytes [32]. It was found that YKL-40 worked synergistically with insulin growth factor-1 (IGF-1) to induce fibroblasts growth [21]. YKL-40 was discussed as a differentiation marker for monocytes [7], mesenchymal stem cells [43], and chondrocytes [44].

YKL-40 functions as a migration and adhesion factor for vascular cells and helps the formation of branching tubules. Thus, the glycoprotein could play a role in angiogenesis [11].

A variety of independent investigations demonstrated that high levels of YKL-40 were related to metastasis and poor survival in different human carcinomas, such as breast cancer [11], colorectal cancer [45], ovarian cancer [46], high-grade glioma [47], and lymphoma [48], suggesting that YKL-40 might serve as a diagnostic, risk assessment, and prognostic biomarker. Other studies indicated that YKL-40 increased also in inflammatory disorders associated with tissue remodeling and destruction [24, 49].

	Population	Serum YKL-40 levels	References
1.	Danish	43	[33]
2.	French	59	[36]
3.	Chinese	61.1	[37]
4.	Bulgarian	84.19	[35]
5.	Japanese	101.7	[38]
6.	Turkish	114	[34]

Table 1. Mean serum YKL-40 levels (ng/ml) in healthy individuals from different populations [39].

http://dx.doi.org/10.5772/66832

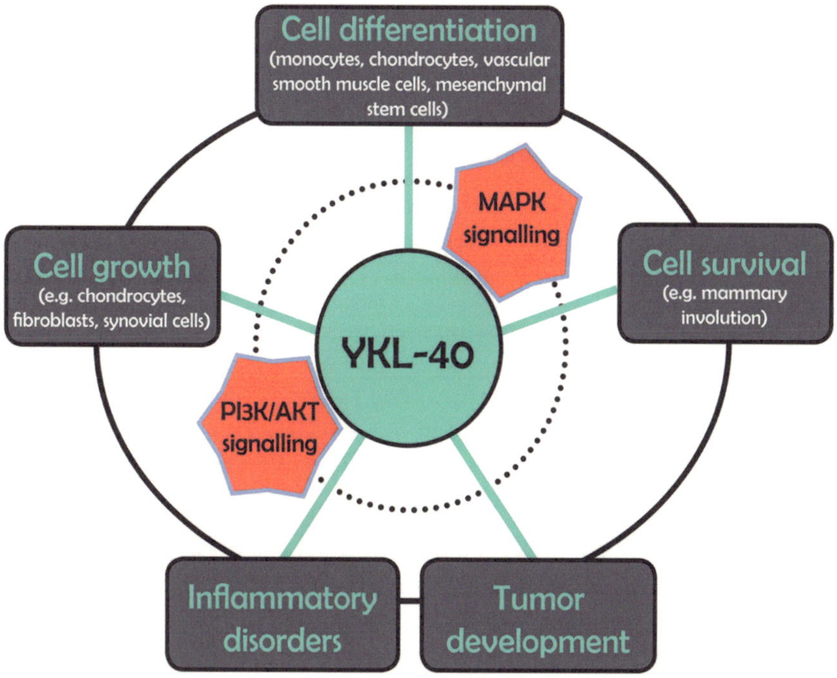

Figure 1. Biological functions of YKL-40. Involvement in cell growth and differentiation, cell survival, inflammatory disorders and tumor development; participation in two basic cell signaling cascades.

YKL-40 is a member of an evolutionary highly conserved protein family, described not only in humans [9, 30], proposing important biological role in normal and pathological conditions. The summarized functions of YKL-40 are presented in **Figure 1**.

3. YKL-40 and rheumatoid arthritis

It is believed that genetic and environmental factors are implicated in the etiology of RA. It is a chronic inflammatory disease which affects about 0.5–1% of the population. Patients suffer from chronic synovial inflammation, joint degradation, and functional disability [50]. Even though some clinical laboratory parameters are related to the risk of radiographic progression, they do not illustrate individual features in the pathogenesis of disease [51].

There is a lack of specific markers for early diagnosis, prognosis, and monitoring of effective treatment. Reliable biomarkers of joint inflammation and destruction in RA should be proteins produced by cells in the synovial fluid and leading to pathological alterations. YKL-40 is expressed and secreted by activated macrophages and neutrophils, fibroblast-like synovial cells, chondrocytes, and vascular smooth muscle cells [32]. Our immunocytochemical study also found that YKL-40 was present in polymorphonuclear cells in the synovial fluid of RA patients [52]. We suppose that it might reflect more precisely the local inflammatory process.

The investigations on the significance of serum YKL-40 as a novel inflammatory biomarker are polar. Some researchers show that it could be useful as an informative parameter in disease diagnosis and monitoring [53], and others state that it is merely a marker of joint inflammation [54].

3.1. YKL-40 in serum and synovial fluid

Johansen detected a 10-fold increase in the concentration of YKL-40 in synovial fluid compared to serum levels in RA patients and proposed that the level of YKL-40 might reflect cartilage degradation and synovial inflammation in RA [32]. These findings are in agreement with other studies, suggesting that YKL-40 is associated with the development of osteoarthritis and should be considered as a potential target for treatment [55].

Our observations focused on YKL-40 in RA patients also found significantly higher glycoprotein concentrations in the synovial fluid in comparison with serum levels [35]. However, we determined the same pattern of expression in other inflammatory joint diseases such as osteoarthritis, gout, and psoriatic arthritis [56].

Huber et al. established synovial antigen microarray technology to analyze antibody profile in RA patients. The synovial glycoprotein YKL-40 was one of the 225 peptides and proteins studied, and it was proved to generate autoantibody production [57]. YKl-40 was also detected as a target of T cells and as a specific and independent histologic marker in arthritic synovitis [58, 59].

There are a number of studies in which a multi-biomarker disease activity (MBDA) score is used to evaluate disease activity, prediction of radiographic progression, and prognosis in RA patients. MBDA score is estimated by measuring the concentrations of 12 serum biomarkers. YKL-40 is a part of the established panel of parameters [60, 61]. This fact confirms the potential significance of YKL-40 in the pathogenic route of RA.

The role of YKL-40 in inflammation still remains to be resolved. The question is whether YKL-40 is an active participant in the process of inflammation or is a result of the body response to it.

3.2. YKL-40 and conventional laboratory parameters

C-reactive protein (CRP) and erythrocyte sedimentation rate (ESR) are the best known and frequently used conventional parameters at the time of diagnosis of RA, but they are not considered as predictors of poor prognosis. Radiological progression of joint destruction could often appear despite normal values. This is a common event in early RA stages [62].

Several studies investigated the significance of YKL-40 in relation to CRP and ESR [53]. We also determined a strong association between YKL-40 levels in serum and synovial fluid and CRP and ESR [35]. Thus, YKL-40 could be regarded as an informative proinflammatory biomarker.

3.3. YKL-40 and ultrasonography

Angiogenesis is a major result of synovial inflammation and maintenance of the pannus in RA [63]. Conventional radiology and tomography could not provide direct visualization of

http://dx.doi.org/10.5772/66832

the joint cartilage. The decreased in joint space is only an indirect evidence for joint destruction. Some authors use ultrasonograhy to measure and register early arthritic changes in joint thickness and to figure joint surfaces before they could be detected by routine radiologic methods [64]. We also applied ultrasonography as a sensitive technique for detecting synovial alteration. A relationship between ultrasonographic findings and YKL-40 was detected. Analysis of the data confirmed that the sonographic inflammation correlated with angiogenesis of the synovial membrane [35].

3.4. YKL-40 and angiogenesis

Vascular epidermal growth factor (VEGF) is a key factor in the pathogenesis of RA, serving both as a cell mitogen for endothelial cells and as a factor defining vascular permeability [65]. Several research groups revealed that secreted and expressed VEGF was related to the inflammatory response, to changes in the synovium, and to other conventional markers [65, 66].

YKL-40 also promotes attachment and migration of vascular endothelial cells, which indicates that the protein participates in angiogenesis [11]. Francescone et al. showed that YKL-40 induced VEGF expression in the U87 glioblastoma cell line and supposed that both molecules synergistically promoted endothelial cell angiogenesis [67].

VEGF was influenced by hypoxia, which contributed to RA development and altered response in arthritic synovium [64]. Similarly, YKL-40 was also upregulated by hypoxia in tumor cells [25]. It is assumed that the pathogenic features of arthritic synovium share the same characteristics with tumor cells.

3.5. YKL-40 and cytokines

Recent studies defined proinflammatory cytokines as major participants in RA pathogenesis resulting in identification of new molecular targets. It was shown that the production of tumor necrosis factor-alpha (TNF-α) is involved in the pathogenesis of RA [68], and biological inhibitors of this cytokine were approved for clinical use [69]. It was proved that levels of proinflammatory cytokines such as IL-1α, TNF-α, IL-6, and IFN-γ in the serum and synovial fluid of RA patients correlated with disease activity and progression [70]. Our investigations determined a strong link between serum and synovial levels of YKL-40 and serum TNF-α and IL-1β in patients with RA [71]. The cellular sources of TNF-α and IL-1β are circulating monocytes and macrophages [72]. It was shown that YKL-40 originated from the same cell types [32].

4. Conclusion

Investigations published so far determine YKL-40 as an important molecule in RA pathogenesis. It is assumed that circulating YKL-40 might reflect precisely the activity of local and systemic inflammation. The clinical utility of YKL-40 as diagnostic or prognostic marker in RA remains to be further clarified, but still it gives rise to serious expectations in the search of new promising biomarkers.

Acknowledgements

The studies are supported by Medical University–Plovdiv—Grants No-01/2009, NO-01/2010, DP-08/2012 and partially by DUNK 01/2009 from the Ministry of Education and Science—Bulgaria.

The authors thank Yana Feodorova, PhD for the help in the design of the figure.

Author details

Maria H. Kazakova and Victoria S. Sarafian*

*Address all correspondence to: victoriasarafian@gmail.com

Department of Medical Biology, Faculty of Medicine, Medical University-Plovdiv, Bulgaria

References

[1] Strimbu K, Tavel J. What are biomarkers? Curr Opin HIV AIDS. 2010;6:463–466. doi:10.1097/COH.0b013e32833ed177

[2] Atkinson AJ. Biomarkers and surrogate endpoints: preferred definitions and conceptual framework. Clin Pharmacol Ther. 2001;69:89–95.

[3] Morrow D, Cannon C, Jesse R, et al. Clinical characteristics and utilization of biochemical markers in acute coronary syndromes. Circulation. 2007;13:356–375.

[4] Hakala B, White C, Recklies AD. Human cartilage gp-39, a major secretory product of articular chondrocytes and synovial cells, is a mammalian member of a chitinase protein family. J Biol Chem. 1993;268:25803–25810.

[5] Chaplin D. Overview of the immune response. J Allergy Clin Immunol. 2010;125:S3–23. doi:10.1016/j.jaci.2009.12.9802012

[6] Johansen JS, Williamson MK, Rice JS, et al. Identification of proteins secreted by human osteoblastic cells in culture. J Bone Miner Res. 1992;7:501–512.

[7] Rehli M, Krause SW, Andreesen R. Molecular characterization of the gene for human cartilage gp-39(CHI3L1), a member of the chitinase protein family and marker for late stages of macrophage differentiation. Genomics. 1997;43:221–225.

[8] Harvey S, Whaley J, Eberhardt K. The relationship between serum levels of YKL-40 and disease progression in patients with early rheumatoid arthritis. Scand J Rheumatol. 2000;29:391–393.

[9] Morrison BW, Leder P. neu and ras initiate murine mammary tumors that share genetic markers generally absent in c-myc and int-2-initiated tumors. Oncogene. 1994;9:3417–3426.

[10] Fusetti F, Pijning T, Kalk KH, Bos E, Dijkstra BW. Crystal structure and carbohydrate-binding properties of the human cartilage glycoprotein-39. J Biol Chem. 2003;278:37753–37760.

[11] Shao R. YKL-40 acts as an angiogenic factor to promote tumor angiogenesis. Front Physiol. 2013;4:122.

[12] McQuade KJ, Beauvais DM, Burbach BJ, Rapraeger AC. Syndecan-1 regulates alphav-beta5 integrin activity in B82L fibroblasts. J Cell Sci. 2006;119:2445–2456.

[13] Faibish M, Francescone R, Bentley B, Yan W, Shao R. A YKL-40-neutralizing antibody blocks tumor angiogenesis and progression: a potential therapeutic agent in cancers. Mol Cancer Ther. 2011;10:742–751. doi:10.1158/1535-7163.MCT-10-0868

[14] Kim H, Lee B, Song Y, et al. Potential association between coronary artery disease and the inflammatory biomarker YKL-40 in asymptomatic patients with type 2 diabetes mellitus. Cardiovasc Diabetol. 2012;11:84. doi:10.1186/1475-2840-11-84

[15] Malemud Ch. Intracellular signaling pathways in rheumatoid arthritis. J Clin Cell Immunol. 2013. doi:10.4172/2155-9899.1000160

[16] Wisler BA, Dennis JE, Malemud CJ. New organ-specific pharmacological strategies interfering with signaling pathways in inflammatory disorders/autoimmune disorders. Curr Signal Transduct Ther. 2011;6:279–291.

[17] Kjaergaard A, Johansen J, Bojesen S, Nordestgaard B. Role of inflammatory marker YKL-40 in the diagnosis, prognosis and cause of cardiovascular and liver diseases. Crit Rev Clin Lab Sci. 2016. doi:10.1080/10408363.2016.1190683

[18] Clarke DN, Al Ahmad A, Lee B, et al. Perlecan domain V induces VEGf secretion in brain endothelial cells through integrin $\alpha5\beta1$ and ERK-dependent signaling pathways. PLoS One. 2012;7:e45257.

[19] Rabinovich D, Croci G. Regulatory circuits mediated by lectin-glycan interactions in autoimmunity and cancer. Immunity. 2012;36:322–335.

[20] He C, Lee CG, Cruz C, Lee CM, Zhou Y,Ahangari F, et al. Chitinase 3-like 1 regulates cellular and tissue responses via IL-13 receptor $\alpha2$. Cell Rep. 2013;4(4):830–841. doi:10.1016/j.celrep.2013.07.032

[21] De Ceuninck F, Gaufillier S, Bonnaud A, Sabatini M, Lesur C, Pastoureau P. YKL-40 (Cartilage gp-39) induces proliferative events in cultured chondrocytes and synoviocytes and increases glycosaminoglycan synthesis in chondrocytes. Biochem Biophys Res Commun. 2001;285:926–931.

[22] Johansen JS, Olee T, Price PA, Hashimoto S, Ochs RL, Lotz M. Regulation of YKL-40 production by human articular chondrocytes. Arthritis Rheum. 2001;44:826–837.

[23] Bonneh-Barkay D, Bissel S, Kofler J, Starkey A, Guoji Wang G, Clayton A. Wiley Astrocyte and macrophage regulation of YKL-40 expression and cellular response in neuroinflammation. Brain Pathol. 2012;22:530–546. doi:10.1111/j.1750-3639.2011.00550.x

[24] Väänänen T, Koskinen A, Paukkeri E, et al. YKL-40 as a novel factor associated with inflammation and catabolic mechanisms in osteoarthritic joints. Mediat Inflamm. 2014. doi:10.1155/2014/215140

[25] Junker N, Johansen JS, Hansen LT, Lund EL, Kristjansen PEG. Regulation of YKL-40 expression during genotoxic or microenvironmental stress in human glioblastoma cells. Cancer Sci. 2005;96:183–190.

[26] Kunz L, Wout E, Schadewijk A, Postma D, Kerstjens, Sterk P, Hiemstra P. Regulation of YKL-40 expression by corticosteroids: effect on pro-inflammatory macrophages in vitro and its modulation in COPD in vivo. Respir. Res. 2015;16:154–164.

[27] Zhang W, Kawanishi M, Miyake K et al. Association between YKL-40 and adult primary astrocytoma. Cancer. 2010;116:2688–2697.

[28] Stokes DG, Liu G, Coimbra IB, Piera-Velazquez S, Crowl RM, Jimenez SA. Assessment of the gene expression profile of differentiated and dedifferentiated human fetal chondrocytes by microarray analysis. Arthritis Rheum. 2002;46:404–419.

[29] Scully S, Yan W, Bentley B, Cao Q, Shao R. Inhibitory activity of YKL-40 in mammary epithelial cell differentiation and polarization induced by lactogenic hormones: a role in mammary tissue involution. PLoS One. 2011;6:e25819. doi:10.1371/journal.pone.0025819

[30] Johansen JS, Høyer PE, Larsen LA, Price PA, Møllgård K. YKL-40 protein expression in the early developing human musculoskeletal system. J Histochem Cytochem. 2007;55:1213–1228.

[31] Bojesen SE, Johansen JS, Nostegaard BG. Plasma YKL-40 levels in healthy subjects from the general population. Clin Chim Acta. 2011. doi:10.1016/j.cca.2011.01.022

[32] Johansen JS. Studies on serum YKL-40 as a biomarker in diseases with inflammation, tissue remodelling, fibroses and cancer. Dan Med Bull. 2006;53:172–209.

[33] Johansen JS, Lottenburger T, Nielsen HJ, Jensen JE, Svendsen MN, Kollerup G, Christensen IJ. Weekly, and long-time variation in serum concentrations of YKL-40 in healthy subjects. Cancer Epidemiol Biomarkers Prev. 2008:2603–2608.

[34] Gungen G, Ardic F, Findikoglu G, Rota S. The effect of mud pack therapy on serum YKL-40 and hsCRP levels in patients with knee osteoarthritis. Rheumatol Int. 2009. doi:10.1007/s00296-010-1727-4

[35] Kazakova M, Batalov A, Deneva T, Mateva N, Kolarov Z, Sarafian V. Relationship between sonographic parameters and YKL-40 levels in rheumatoid arthritis. Rheumatol Int. 2013;33:341–346.

[36] Conrozier Th, Carlier M-C, Mathieu P, Colson F, Debard AL, Richard S, et al. Serum levels of YKL-40 and C reactive protein in patients with hip osteoarthritis and healthy subjects: a cross sectional study. Ann Rheum Dis. 2000;59:828–831.

[37] Zou X, Zhang W. The efficacy of YKL-40 and CA125 as biomarkers for epithelial ovarian cancer. Braz J Med Biol Res. 2010;43:1232–1238.

[38] Yamamori H, Hashimoto R, Ohi K, Yasuda Y, Fukumoto M, Kasahara E, et al. A promoter variant in the chitinase 3-like 1 gene is associated with serum YKL-40 level and personality trait. Neurosci Lett. 2012;513:204–208.

[39] Kazakova M, Sarafian V. YKL-40 in health and disease: a challenge for joint inflammation. Biomed Rev. 2013;24:49–56.

[40] Ling H, Recklies AD. The chitinase 3-like protein human cartilage glycoproein 39 inhibits cellular responses to the inflammatory cytokines interleukin-1 and tumor necrosis factor-alpha. Biochem J. 2004;380:651–659.

[41] Malinda KM, Ponce L, Kleinman HK, et al. Gp38k, a protein synthesized by vascular smooth muscle cells, stimulates directional migration of human umbilical vein endothelial cells. Exp Cell Res 1999;250:168–173.

[42] Lee CG, Hartl D, Lee GR, Koller B, Matsuura H, Da Silva CA, Sohn MH, Cohn L, Homer RJ, Kozhich AA, et al. Role of breast regression protein 39 (BRP-39)/chitinase 3-like-1 in Th2 and IL-13-induced tissue responses and apoptosis. J Exp Med. 2009;206:1149–1166.

[43] Hoover D, Zhu V, Chen R, Briley, Rameshwar P, et al. Expression of the chitinase family glycoprotein YKL-40 in undifferentiated, differentiated and trans-differentiated mesenchymal stem cells. PLoS One. 2013;8. doi:info:doi/10.1371/journal.pone.0096230

[44] Imabayashi H, Mori T, Gojo S, Kioyono T, Sugiyama T, Irie R, Isoga T, Hata J, Toyama Y, Umezawa A. Redifferentiation of dedifferentiated chondrocytes and chondrogenesis of human bone marrow stromal cells via chondrosphere formation with expression profiling by large-scale cDNA analysis. Exp Cell Res 2003;288:35–50.

[45] Johansen JS, Christensen IJ, Jørgensen L, Olsen J, Rahr H, Nielsen K, Laurberg S, Brünner N, Nielsen H. Serum YKL-40 in risk assessment for colorectal cancer: a prospective study of 4,496 subjects at risk of colorectal cancer. Cancer Epidemiol Biomarkers Prev. 2015;3:621–626. doi:10.1158/1055-9965.EPI-13-1281

[46] Chiang YC, Lin HW, Chang CF, Chang MC, Fu CF, Chen TC, et al. Overexpression of CHI3L1 is associated with chemoresistance and poor outcome of epithelial ovarian carcinoma. Oncotarget. 2015;6:39740–39755.

[47] Steponaitis G, Skiriute D, Kazlauskas A, Golubickaite I, Stakaitis R, Tamašauskas A, Vaitkiene P. High CHI3L1 expression is associated with glioma patient survival. Diagn Pathol. 2016;11:42. doi:10.1186/s13000-016-0492-4

[48] Hottinger A, Iwamoto F, Karimi S, Riedel E, Dantis J, Park J, et al. YKL-40 and MMP-9 as serum markers for patients with primary central nervous system lymphoma. Ann Neurol. 2011;70:163–169. doi:10.1002/ana.22360

[49] Létuvé S, Kozhich A, Arouche N, Grandsaigne M, Reed J, Dombret MC, et al. YKL-40 is elevated in patients with chronic obstructive pulmonary disease and activates alveolar macrophages. J Immunol. 2008;181:5167–5173.

[50] Mclnnes I, Schett G. The pathogenesis of rheumatoid arthritis. N Engl J Med. 2011;365:2205-2219.

[51] Liao KP, Weinblatt ME, Cui J, et al. Clinical predictors of erosion-free status in rheumatoid arthritis: a prospective cohort study. Rheumatology (Oxford). 2011;50:1473–1479.

[52] Kazakova M, Batalov A, Kolarov Z, Sarafian V. Serum and synovial YKL-40 levels in psoriatic arthritis. Sci Technnol. 2012;2:60–63.

[53] Kassem I, Mahmoud L, Salah W. Study of resistin and YKL-40 in rheumatoid arthritis. J Am Sci. 2010;6:1004–1012.

[54] Syversen SW, Goll GL, Heijde D, Landeve R, Lie BA, Odegard S, et al. Prediction of radiographic progression in rheumatoid arthritis and the role of antibodies against mutated citrullinated vimentin: results from a 10-year prospective study. Ann Rheum Dis. 2009;69:345–351. doi:10.1136/ard.2009.113092

[55] Szychlinska M, Trovato F, Di Rosa M, Malaguarnera L, Puzzo L, Leonardi R, Castrogiovanni P, Musumeci G. Co-expression and co-localization of cartilage glycoproteins CHI3L1 and lubricin in osteoarthritic cartilage: morphological, immunohistochemical and gene expression profiles. Int J Mol Sci. 2016:17:359. doi:10.3390/ijms17030359

[56] Kazakova M, Batalov A, Mateva N, Kolarov Z, Sarafian V. Comparative significance of YKL-40 in different types of arthritis. In: Front. Immunol. Conference 15th International Congress of Immunology (ICI); 22-28 August 2013; Milan. Italy: doi:10.3389/conf.fiL

[57] Hueber W, Kidd B, Tomooka B, Lee B, Bruce B, Fries J, et al. Antigen microarray profiling of autoantibodies in rheumatoid arthritis. Arthritis Rheum. 2005;52:2645–2655. doi::10.1002/art.21269

[58] Cope A, Sonderstrup G. Evaluating candidate autoantigens in rheumatoid arthritis. Springer Semin Immunopathol. 1998;20:23–39.

[59] Baeten D, Steenbakkers PG, Rijnders AM, Boots AM, Veys EM, de Keyser F. Detection of major histocompatibility complex/human cartilage gp-39 complexes in rheumatoid arthritis synovitis as a specific and independent histologic marker. Arthritis Rheum. 2004;50:444–451.

[60] Bakker M, Cavet G, WG Jacobs J, Bijlsma J, Haneym D, Shen Y, Hesterberg L, et al. Performance of a multi-biomarker score measuring rheumatoid arthritis disease activity in the CAMERA tight control study. Ann Rheum Dis. 2012;71:1692–1697.

[61] Hambardzumyan K, Bolce R, Saevarsdottir S, Cruickshank S, Sasso E, et al. Pretreatment multi-biomarker disease activity score and radiographic progression in early RA: results from the SWEFOT trial. Ann Rheum Dis. 2015;74:1102–1109.

[62] Emery P, Salmon M. Early rheumatoid arthritis: time to aim for remission? Ann Rheum Dis. 1995;54:944–947.

[63] Paleolog E. The vasculature in rheumatoid arthritis: cause or consequence? Int J Exp Pathol. 2009;90:249–261.

[64] Batalov A, Kuzmanova S, Penev D. Ultrasonographic evaluation of knee joint cartilage in rheumatoid arthritis patients. Folia Med. 2000;4:23–26.

[65] Lee S, Joo Y, Kim W, et al. Vascular endothelial growth factor levels in the serum and synovial fluid of patients with rheumatoid arthritis. Clin Exp Rheumatol. 2001;19:321–324.

[66] Sone H, Sakauchi M, Takahashi A, et al. Elevated levels of vascular endothelial growth factor in the sera of patients with rheumatoid arthritis correlation with disease activity. Life Sci. 2001;69:1861–1869.

[67] Francescone RA, Scully S, Faibish M, et al. Role of YKL-40 in the angiogenesis, radioresistance, and progression og glioblastoma. J Biol Chem. 2011. doi:10.1074/jbc.M110.212514

[68] Feldmann M, Maini R. Discovery of TNF-alpha as a therapeutic target in rheumatoid arthritis: preclinical and clinical studies. Joint Bone Spine. 2002;69:12–18.

[69] Maini R, Taylor P. Anti-cytokine therapy for rheumatoid arthritis. Annu Rev Med. 2000;51:207–229.

[70] Kolarov Z, Altunkova I, Baleva M, Martinova F, Monov S, Shumnalieva R. Relation between serum and synovial fluei levels of IL-1-alpha, TNF-alpha, IL-6, IFN-gamma and sIL-6r and clinical, immunological and genetic factors in rheumatoid arthritis patients. In: Ann. Rheum. Dis Annual European Congress of Rheumatol. EULAR 2015; 10-13 June 2015; Italy: p. 914.

[71] Kazakova-Velinova M. Immunobiological studies on YKL-40 in inflammatory joint and tumor processes [PhD thesis]. Medical University, Plovdiv; 2013.

[72] Arleevskaya M, Gabdoulkhakova A, Filina J, et al. Mononuclear phagocytes in rheumatoid arthritis patients and their relatives-family similarity. Open Rheumatol J. 2011;5:36–44.